Living Life Free From Pain
Treating Arthritis, Joint Pain, Muscle Pain and Fibromyalgia with Maharishi Ayurveda

About the Author

Dr Kumuda Reddy has been practicing medicine for nearly forty years. She has developed a very informative website called "allhealthyfamily.com" which is dedicated to bringing the knowledge of the unlimited scope of Maharishi Ayurvedic Medicine. It is comprehensive, holistic and compatible with Conventional medicine.

Dr Reddy completed her residency and fellowship at Mt.Sinai Hospital, New York. She was the Medical Director of Maharishi Vedic Center in Bethesda, Maryland and a former faculty member of Albany Medical College. She was the Medical Director of Maharishi Rejuvenation Center in Thailand and travels extensively offering consultations across the globe.

Dr. Reddy, through her practice, books and lectures conveys this simple message, "that we are one with nature." Because of our intimate connection to nature and the entire cosmos, we need natural and holistic medicine. It is the need of our time. No other medicine has proven to be as natural, comprehensive, time-tested and holistic as Maharishi Ayurveda.

Dr. Reddy believes that the best way to avoid suffering and ill-health is to "avert the danger which has not yet come." This is the basic principle of prevention from the ancient Vedic tradition of health care. The earlier we start the better.

Taking this to heart, Dr. Reddy has co-authored several books.

Forever Healthy – Introduction to Maharishi Ayur-Veda Health Care
For a Blissful Baby – Healthy and Happy Pregnancy with Maharishi Vedic Medicine
Conquering Chronic Disease – Through Maharishi Vedic Medicine
Golden Transition – Menopause Made Easy
Ayurvedic cooking made easy – 100+ recipes for a healthy YOU

Dr. Reddy has also co-authored a book of stories from the Upanishads entitled "All Love Flows to the Self – Eternal Stories from the Upanishads" and a series of children's stories called the Timeless Wisdom series based on traditional Indian stories that she first heard from her grandmother. Dr. Reddy believes these stories will help educate children in the positive, nourishing and practical values that are so important for their health and happiness.

She has appeared on several radio and TV shows. Dr. Reddy has been contributing health articles to the local news magazines and papers. In addition to her life as a medical doctor, writer and speaker, Dr. Reddy is a wife, mother and an active community leader.

At your bookstore or from the publisher:
Samhita Productions
College Park, Maryland
www.allhealthyfamily.com

Living Life Free From Pain
Treating Arthritis, Joint Pain, Muscle Pain and Fibromyalgia
with Maharishi Ayurveda

by

Kumuda Reddy, M.D.
With Cynthia Lane

Published by
Samhita Productions
College Park, Maryland

© 2002 by Maharishi Vedic Education Development Corporation and Kumuda Readdy, M.D. All rights reserved. No part of this book may be reproduced or transmitted in any form or by any means, electronic or mechanical, including photocopying, recording, or by any information storage and retrieval system, without permission in writing from the author and publisher.

©Maharishi Vedic Medicine, Maharishi Sthapatya veda, Maharishi Jyotish, transcendental Meditation, TM, Maharishi Transcendental Meditation, TM-Sidhi, Maharishi Vedic Approach to Health, Maharishi Vedic Astrology, Maharishi Yoga, Maharishi Ayur-Veda, maharishi Ayur-Veda Health Center, Maharishi Rejuvenation, Maharishi Amrit kalash, maharishi Rasayana program, and maharishi Vedic Science are registered or common law trademarks licensed to Maharishi Vedic Education Development corporation and used with permission. Genitrack and Therapecutic Aroma are trademarks of Maharishi Ayur-Veda products International.

Book Design and Composition - Pixint (www.pixint.com)

Printed in the United States of America.

ISBN- 1-4392-3795-6

Dedication

To Maharishi Mahesh Yogi, for giving us his vision of natural and holistic health in all areas of our lives.

Acknowledgments

We would like to thank His Majesty Raja Ram, His Excellency Keith Wallace, Samantha Wallace, Dr. Edwards Smith, Vaidya Hemant Gupta, Catherine Peckman, Mary Zielback, Martha Bright, Sandra Willbanks, Shyamala Narayanan, Pixint Group and many others in the production of this book.

Contents

Foreword _____ xv
Chapter 1 - Health and the Big Picture _____ 1
    The USA: Number One in Degenerative Diseases _____ 4
    The Ayurvedic Option _____ 5
    A Little Bit of Medical History: How the Mind and Body Got Conceptually Separated _____ 6
    Carol's Story _____ 9
    Hippocrates _____ 12
Chapter 2 - Joint Disease: Living in the Kingdom of Aches and Painsy ___ 15
    Arthritis _____ 15
    Our Brilliantly-Engineered Joints _____ 17
    Rheumatoid Arthritis _____ 18
    Osteoarthritis: Losing Our Natural Shock-Absorbers _____ 21
    Fibromyalgia: Pain All Over _____ 24
    Lupus _____ 26
    Gout: How Can A Toe Hurt So Much? _____ 29
    Ankylosing Spondylitis: The Stiff Spine _____ 31
    Repetitive Motion and Disease: Carpal Tunnel Syndrome _____ 32
    Had Enough? _____ 34
Chapter 3 - The Miracle of Human Life _____ 37
    Intelligence is Everywhere _____ 38
    Our Dazzling Nervous System _____ 39
    DNA: Our Central Intelligence Agency _____ 41
Chapter 4 - What is Maharishi Vedic Medicine? _____ 45
    What is Maharishi Vedic Medicine? _____ 45
    Comprehensive Healing _____ 46
    The Managing Intelligence of the Universe _____ 47
    Veda 101 _____ 50
    The Primary Cause of Disease _____ 52
    Universal Patterns of Orderliness _____ 54

Chapter 5 - The Components of Balance: Template for a Pain-Free Life Page 57
    Ayurvedic Anatomy _____58
    The Three Mental Qualities _____60
    The Five Elements _____64
    Doshas: The Fundamentals of Balance _____66
    The Doshas in Detail _____69
    Mary's Story _____78
    The Doshic Stages of Life _____80
    The Doshas Are Everywhere _____82
    The Doshas and the Daily Cycle _____82
    The Doshas and the Seasonal Cycle _____83
    The Doshas and the Digestive Cycle _____84
    The Transcendental Meditation® (TM®) Technique _____84

Chapter 6 Digestion: The Pivotal Process _____89
    The Seven Sequential Tissues _____92
    Ama: Gumming Up the Works _____94
    The Srotas: A System for Communicating and Getting Around _____95
    Ama and the Doshas _____100
    Ama, Digestion and Disease _____100
    Ojas and Arthritis _____103
    Creating and Maintaining Ojas _____104

Chapter 7 An Ayurvedic Portrait of Arthritis _____107
    Ayurveda and the Path of Disease _____107
    Marilyn: A Case Study in Osteoarthritis _____108
    Hindsight _____109
    The Six Stages of Disease _____110
    Taking It All Down to the Doshas _____116
    Ankylosing Spondylitis _____118
    Ama, Vata and Fibromyalgia (Ama Rasa) _____119
    Amavata: Rheumatoid Arthritis _____122
    Lupus _____124
    Helping Karen Deal with Lupus _____125
    Vata Rakta: Gouty Arthritis _____126
    Carpal Tunnel Syndrome _____128

Chapter 8 - Food and Freedom from Joint Disease   **131**
   The Two Phases of Digestion   131
   The Three Forms of Taste   133
   The Six Tastes and Digestion   134
   Examples of Six Tastes   135
   Food and Arthritis: Making Intelligent Choices   136
   A Few More Facts about Food   138
   The Qualities of Food Based on the Doshas   139
   Potency   140
   The Mental Effects of Food   141

Chapter 9 - Holding Health in Your Hands   **157**
   Daily and Seasonal Routines: Flowing with Natural Cycles   159
   FMS and a Healthy Routine   161
   Speech, Action and Illness   166
   Maharishi Rejuvenation Therapy (MRT)   169
   Three Stages of Treatment   171
   The TM-Sidhi® Program   176

Chapter 10 - Herbs and Rasayanas: Healing Gifts From the Plant Kingdom   **179**
   Herbal Compounds: Creating Wholeness   181
   Choosing the Right Herbal Formula   183
   Herbs for Arthritis   183
   Medicated Oils   185
   Aroma Therapy   186
   Rasayanas   187

Chapter 11 - Ever-Increasing Possibilities   **189**
   Healing with Sound Maharishi Vedic Vibration Technology   189
   Instant Relief from Arthritis   191
   Maharishi Gandharva Veda   192
   Maharishi Yoga Asanas   193
   Pranayama: Neurorespiratory Therapy   194
   Maharishi Vedic Architecture: Sthapatya Veda   195

Chapter 12 - Prevention   **201**
   The Amazing Art of Nadi Vigyan   201
   Personal Preventive Measures   204

Maharishi Jyotish: Averting Danger Before It Arises _____ 206
Chapter 13 - Pulling Everything Together: The End of This Book and Joint Disease _____ **211**
    Additional Recommendations _____ 215
    In Case You Still Have Questions _____ 217
    Ayurveda: A Compassionate Science _____ 221
Index _____ **225**
Appendix: Resources _____ **231**

Foreward

As a young rheumatologist in private practice, I began to develop symptoms of arthritis. My grandmother was crippled by rheumatoid arthritis, and I remembered both her pain and the promise that I made to her to find a solution to this agonizing disease. The suffering of my grandmother as well as thousands of my patients was all too clear in my mind and I frankly felt terrified. Of course, I ran a full panel of laboratory tests. They all came back negative, in spite of the pain in my hips and the small joints of my hands as well as small collections of fluid in my knees when I exercised.

As the dust settled, I gradually realized that the pattern of my complaints best fit osteoarthritis. This meant that my joint problems would most likely come and go except for chronic low back pain that was the result of an injury incurred several years earlier. About two years later, I happened to learn the Transcendental Meditation® (TM®) technique. Many aspects of my health soon improved, but my joint problems continued to wax and wane. After meditating a while longer, I spontaneously improved my diet and my joints then also got better. Only the pesky back pain remained.

I was so impressed with the changes that resulted from my TM practice that I started encouraging my patients to learn. For ten years I observed that my meditating patients did far better than those who had not learned and I decided to pursue this direction full time. I quit my practice and joined the faculty at Maharishi University of Management (MUM) in Fairfield, Iowa. I was trained in Maharishi Vedic Medicine and began to consult regularly with Vedic physicians. I experienced just about all the treatments that Dr. Kumuda Reddy has outlined in this wonderful book.

I remember asking a leading expert in Vedic medicine from India whether he felt that anything could be done for the chronic back pain from my sixteen-year-old injury. It still bothered me and competent Western physicians had recommended back surgery. The Vedic doctor shook his head from side to side and said, "We can try." I thought that I was getting a double message, until I learned that in India, shaking your head from side to side doesn't mean "no." It can actually be an expression of enthusiasm.

Over the next few years, I followed this doctor's advice, as well as that of a number of others who followed him. One day I realized that I had not felt any back pain for some time. To this day, ten years later, I continue to be free of the pain that had been a regular feature of my life for sixteen years. My other joint problems have also diminished. These days they only raise their heads if I go off my good routine. When I add this to the experiences of my patients who use Maharishi Vedic Medicine, I feel that I have fulfilled my promise to my grandmother.

I advise you to read this succinct and coherent book carefully. Dr. Reddy's skillfully composed work on the treatment of arthritis-and even more importantly, its prevention-shows us that contrary to what we may hear from contemporary medicine, arthritis is not incurable and its cause is not unknown. Though not widely appreciated in the West, Vedic medicine has known about both the cause of arthritis and its treatment all along.

When arthritis is far advanced, it is not easy to cure , but let me share with you the experience of two female patients in their mid-thirties. They both had the clinical signs of early onset rheumatoid arthritis, complete with hot, swollen joints, multiple joint involvement and morning stiffness. Their symptoms had been present for more than three months. I placed them on a Maharishi Vedic Medicine protocol that included instructions for diet, daily routine and herbs. When I met with them again after several months, I asked whether they had taken the recommended herbs and how they were doing. I asked about the herbs first because I had not completely shed my reliance on "medicines."

As it turned out, neither of the women had gotten the herbs, but they had followed the dietary and behavioral recommendations and felt "just fine." When I examined them, I found that their joints were no longer red, hot and swollen. Four years later they still remained free of joint pain and swelling. As you can imagine, I was delighted. In all my years of practicing rheumatology, I had never been accused of curing anyone of rheumatoid arthritis.

I find the idea of preventing arthritis even more exciting than the cure. Here in the West, we need to recognize that disease is neither capricious nor malicious. Our health, or lack of it, is the product of our own doing. To quote Pogo, "We have met the enemy and they are us." Dr. Reddy has given us the knowledge of how to make peace with ourselves and spare ourselves from debilitating illness.

My personal experience, research and work with patients all confirm the value and validity of what Dr. Reddy offers in this small volume. She did not invent this information. It has been there for thousands of years. However, she has performed a tremendous service by extracting it from multiple sources and giving us a concise rendering of information that is going to revolutionize the approach to arthritis in the West. I know my grandmother would be very happy.

Dr. Edwards Smith, MD. FACP
Dean, Maharishi College of Vedic Medicine
Albuquerque, New Mexico,
September, 2000

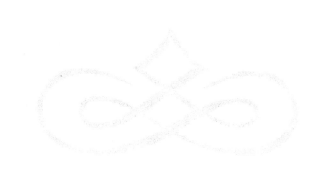

CHAPTER 1

Health and the Big Picture

The range of health includes all areas of individual life, national life, international life, life of the whole world, and Cosmic life. The individual is always a Cosmic Reality-physically, the individual has a Cosmic Physiology, and mentally, the individual has a Cosmic Psychology.[1]

Maharishi Mahesh Yogi

These words open our awareness to a sense of health which is infinitely vast. Just for a moment, we feel expansive, inspired. Something deep inside reverberates with this possibility, this truth, and says, "Yes!"

However, many of us do not yet experience this expansiveness in any consistent way. We do not yet recognize ourselves as cosmic. Our current day-to-day reality may in fact feel full of limitations. Most people, especially those in middle age, expect that advancing years will bring at least some degree of physical limitation and discomfort. It is what we observed in our parents and grandparents, and medical statistics support this expectation. For instance, Americans spend $66 billion each year just to combat headaches.

Of all our health concerns in America, joint problems lead the way. One in three adults has arthritis. As many as one in three families

---

[1] Maharishi Mahesh Yogi, Maharishi Forum of Natural Law and zNational Law for Doctors, Age of Enlightenment Publications, India, 1995, p. 305.

Health and the Big Picture

have to deal with some form of joint condition. Five million Americans suffer from fibromyalgia,[2] and fifty-five million people, or more than eighty percent of those over fifty-five, have osteoarthritis. The American Arthritis Foundation claims that unhealthy joints cost the American economy close to $55 billion annually due to direct medical costs and lost productivity.

According to one author, as many as ninety percent of us will experience osteoarthritis in our Lifetimes[3]. That is virtually an epidemic.

Pain is a regular feature of many people's lives, and if you picked up this book, you are probably familiar with it. If you are fortunate enough to be largely free of pain in your own life, you most likely know someone close to you who is not. If you have an ache here or there, you may have wondered if it is an isolated incident, or if it is leading to something more serious: What would the costs be in terms of limitations on lifestyle? What would you pay psychologically and materially? If pain is a regular feature of your life, then you already know the cost, and how pervasively sickness can influence personal, professional and financial life, both your own and those of family members.

Arthritis is the number one medical problem in the world, but because it is usually non-fatal, it attracts little media coverage and less research than cancer, HIV and heart disease. It is a complex Illness

---

2 Fransen, J., R.N., and Russell, I.J., M.D., Ph.D., The Fibromyalgia Help Book, Smith House Press, Saint Paul, MN, 1966, p. 1.
3 Bucci, L., Ph.D., Pain Free, The Summit Group, Ft. Worth, TX, 1995, pp. 8-9.

with many potential symptoms. Actually, arthritis is a family of diseases, consisting of more than a hundred different conditions. Though a number of drugs and natural therapies are available to reduce pain and mediate other uncomfortable features, no actual medical cure is in sight. This is discouraging for doctors and potentially devastating for patients.

What if it were possible not only to cure these conditions which create such widespread and long-term suffering but also to actually prevent them? What if we could remodel our expectations to encompass a future of greater and greater fulfillment, rather than increasing levels of debilitation? Both my personal experience and my work as a physician with hundreds of patients over the last ten years has shown me that we can and should expect much more of life. I no longer have any doubt that we were born to enjoy genuine health—a state which does far more than preclude pain and disease.

The confidence that I have acquired in using Maharishi Ayurveda over the years is spontaneously conveyed to my patients. Some patients certainly choose Ayurveda as a last resort. Individuals with some form of arthritis or FMS sometimes come to see me after a long history of increasing pain and proliferating secondary symptoms. Their doctors-both the compassionate and frustrated-see little or no hope for restoring health and the patients feel condemned to a lifetime of painkillers. I am so grateful to be able to offer them a truly effective healthcare system. My certainty about this system ignites their optimism and motivates them to participate in their own healing process. Moreover, I am able to share a completely new vision of health with them. The Ayurvedic picture of health incorporates an inner state of deep and ubiquitous happiness and a clear experience of our fundamental connectedness to the totality of life on our planet, in our galaxy and the whole universe.

The USA:

Number One in Degenerative Diseases

Despite the advances made by allopathic healthcare in such areas as diagnostic technologies, the treatment of acute trauma, critical care and the prevention of epidemics; and despite the billions of dollars spent by Americans on conventional medical treatments each year, the United States leads the world in the occurrence of degenerative diseases-arthritis among them. Consequently, many people are searching for other options.

"Our health care system is primarily a disease care system. Last year $2.1 trillion was spent in the U.S. on medical care, 17% of the gross national product. Of these trillions, 95 cents of every dollar was spent to treat disease after it had already occurred."

'Alternative' Medicine Is Mainstream, The Wall Street Journal, January 9, 2009

A 1993 survey in the New England Journal of Medicine offered some information that startled many physicians: Approximately one in three patients used some sort of alternative healthcare in addition to the conventional care provided by the doctors. Seven out of ten did not tell their doctors that they were exploring other options. At the time of the survey, Americans were spending over ten billion dollars on alternatives to allopathic medicine. This amount continues to increase. Clearly, we are looking for medical approaches that incorporate prevention and are based on a comprehensive understanding of health.

The Ayurvedic Option

Ayurvedic medicine is one of the options now being widely explored. In this book, I am going to describe the Ayurvedic system of medicine and its applications to preventing and healing arthritis. Ayurveda is at least 5000 years old, and it is the oldest system of natural medicine still in use. In fact, it had a marked influence on ancient Greek medicine and the Hippocratic tradition, which provided a foundation for allopathic medicine.

The past ten years have brought a proliferation of books on Ayurveda, and the availability of its herbal formulas and other types of treatment in the West has grown substantially. Despite the expanding interest in Ayurveda, however, most people have only a limited understanding of the full range of its perspective on health and its applications to specific diseases. Over time-but especially during the British occupation of India-much of the Vedic knowledge, including Ayurveda, has become fragmented or obscure. Some has been lost completely. Since the early 1980s, Maharishi Mahesh Yogi, founder of the Transcendental Meditation® (TM®) program, has worked with the leading Ayurvedic physicians (vaidyas) of India to restore the Ayurvedic system to its highest level of effectiveness and to make it available throughout the world. Through

Maharishi's efforts and remarkable insights, the most comprehensive and powerful values of Ayurveda have been restored.

Maharishi's Vedic Approach to Health (MVAH)-also called Maharishi Vedic Medicine (MVM)-carries the promise of lasting health and fulfillment. It defines health as wholeness, as do many natural and ancient medical systems. Even conventional medicine is slowly moving away from a biomechanical model for health. Alongside the proliferation of hi-tech treatment modalities and diagnostic equipment, modern doctors are rediscovering the importance of treating the patient, not simply the disease. In Ayurveda, health is not just the absence of disease, but a balanced and vital condition of the whole human system.

A Little Bit of Medical History:

How the Mind and Body Got Conceptually Separated

Today, we hear more and more about the connectedness of mind and body. Medical science is now able to explain the chemistry of this inextricably intimate relationship and we will discuss this in some detail later when we look at the relationship between stress, emotions and the immune system and the development of such diseases as rheumatoid arthritis.[4] However, in becoming aware of the deep interdependency of mind and body, we are only recovering a basic understanding of life that we lost in the West in the early 1600's.

The separation of mind and body in Western medical science and in

---

4 See Chapter Three on the immune system.

the popular understanding of human life began around 1616. An Englishman named Andrew Harvey gave a lecture on blood circulation that triggered a series of events and discoveries that led to a mechanized or biomechanical view of human physiology. In the quest for reliable, genuinely scientific knowledge, information gained through the senses lost its credibility. Increasingly, truth in medicine had to be proved through a rigorous system of experimentation and observation, and there was no place for the consideration of subjective factors, such as the relationship between health and personality, spirituality or inner balance.

The evolving paradigm of the human body as a complex but predictable machine, was strongly reinforced by the seventeenth-century philosopher René Descartes. To resolve a territorial conflict with the Roman Catholic Church and be free to pursue objective science, Descartes declared mind and body to be distinct. The mind, according to Descartes, was non-material, capable of reflecting divine intelligence and of learning and evolving. It remained under the dominion of the Church, in the domain of spirit.

The body, on the other hand, was defined as a concrete entity that functioned automatically. It would maintain its operations even when not directed by the mind. The body was an engine whose parts could be studied and became the domain of science. With this view of the body, Descartes was able to bequeath a research methodology called "reductionism" to science: To understand something complex, reduce it to simpler components and study each one. Reductionism dominated medical research for several centuries and was the basis for many important breakthroughs in understanding how the body's complex systems function and the nature of certain diseases.

France provided another advance in medical science through the work of Louis Pasteur and Robert Koch-the theory of specific etiology. This theory holds that every disease is caused by an identifiable micro-organism. Spectacular breakthroughs resulted from the applications of specific etiology. Dozens of serious and widespread conditions, such as tuberculosis, polio, meningitis and smallpox, were brought under control. However, the success of this approach gave rise to an intense focus on the nature of disease and the treatment of discrete symptoms at the cost of understanding the patient and what creates health. As a result, Western medicine has lost insight (and sometimes even interest) in some critical areas of health. For instance, nothing in allopathy clearly explains why some people get sick while others don't when exposed to the same set of conditions, including specific microorganisms. In addition, the primary causes of many chronic illnesses with highly diverse symptoms, including fibromyalgia and arthritis, remain unknown.

Though medical science has made some amazing achievements in the treatment of disease, the current paradigm faces major challenges. Modern Western medicine has virtually eliminated the human factor in healthcare and largely alienated patients from their physicians. Perhaps most significantly, healing has become something that other people or machines or chemicals do for us. We have forgotten the vast healing power of nature and diminished our ability to access and enliven it.

Many of the patients with arthritic symptoms, who have come to me for help, have felt depressed and hopeless due to the inability of conventional medicine to address their conditions. Many have felt worse due to their sensitivity to prescribed medicines. Some had even been diagnosed as hypochondriacs. All felt significantly better within one to three months after applying the recommendations from Maharishi Vedic Medicine. They also felt more in control of their lives and their health as a result of the increased understanding of the relationship between diet, lifestyle and health which Maharishi Ayurveda provides.

Carol's Story

One such patient was Carol, who came to me for help after hearing me speak about menopause on TV. Carol was in the middle of menopause, but that was just a fraction of her problems. She was a fifty-year-old wife and mother, who also managed her own restaurant. A naturally lively person, when Carol first came to my office, she looked utterly weary as a result of dealing with a great range of uncomfortable symptoms. She had joint pain, mainly in her knee, but also had some pain in her lower back and neck and in the joints of her right hand. Over the years, her digestion and elimination had degenerated. She had constipation, gas and bloating and fluid accumulation in her feet and legs. Carol could not digest any raw vegetables or fruit, and had been told that she had low blood sugar. To top things off, she was depressed and dizzy and had headaches and congested sinuses.

As all these problems piled up, Carol started to feel that life was unbearably stressful. She had been tested for rheumatoid arthritis, but the results were negative. She had had a hysterectomy one year earlier and was now taking a hormone replacement drug. She noted that her fluid retention and digestive problems were aggravated after the surgery, but had started several years before it. She was at a point in her life where she was willing to try anything that would help.

I gave Carol a thorough examination. Using Maharishi Vedic Medicine's precise and comprehensive diagnostic tools, I was able to detect the fundamental causes of her varied symptoms. I prescribed an individualized diet, several herbal formulas and a daily oil massage, to recreate balance at the deepest level of her physiology. Normally, I would also have given her several yoga postures specific to her condition, but she couldn't do them because of joint pain and fluid-related swelling. I suggested that she walk instead.

After one month on her MVM regimen, Carol returned to my office for a check-up. She was less depressed, more alert and her dizziness was gone. Her constipation had improved, she had more energy and some of the joint pain had decreased. After the second month using Maharishi Ayurveda, her headaches had become rare, but she still experienced fluid retention as a result of her hormone prescription. When Carol's other doctors stopped the prescription, her hot flashes became worse. I gave her an MVM regimen for the hot flashes and over the next six weeks, they died down and the fluid retention almost disappeared. By this time, her constipation, sinus problems and headaches were also almost completely gone and joint pains were minimal. I continued to see Carol over the next three or four months, and we focused on strengthening and balancing her digestion and elimination as well as her reproductive system to prevent hot flashes and make menopause a smooth process. After two months, her joint pain was totally gone, except for a rare bout of morning stiffness.

I still see Carol every few months, and she is maintaining her MVM diet and routine. She has returned to full participation in lifeworking, taking care of her family, enjoying her grandchildren.

Carol's perspective has changed as dramatically as her health. In Maharishi Vedic Medicine, we provide a great deal of patient education. Personalized diet and lifestyle recommendations help patients take control of their health and maintain it. Carol now knows the many ways in which she can take charge of her mental and physical well-being. This also helped Carol overcome fears about aging, which stemmed from watching her parents go through a lot of sickness. This book will look at certain diseases affecting the musculoskeletal system, all of which produce chronic pain: osteo- and rheumatoid arthritis, fibromyalgia syndrome, ankylosing spondylitis, gout, systemic lupus erythematosus and carpal tunnel syndrome. Conventional medicine has provided a number of ways to combat the symptoms associated with these conditions, especially pain. These include both complex pharmaceuticals with potent side effects and relatively simple lifestyle recommendations, such as specific forms of exercise and diet. However, both a cure and a complete understanding of the causes elude medical science. It may be necessary to understand the real nature of health and the human healing system to deal effectively with these diseases. To do this,

Western medicine may have to go back to its roots and discover what it has forgotten in its fascination with the engine"s individual elements and systems: The whole is greater than the sum of its parts.

Hippocrates

Natural forces within us are the true healers of disease . . . Health depends on a state of equilibrium among the various factors that govern the operation of the body and the mind; the equilibrium in turn is reached only when man lives in harmony with his external environment.[5]

Hippocrates lived from about 460-377 B.C. on the Greek island of Kos, and is considered to be the founder of Western medicine and the first proponent for the rational study of disease. He and his followers tried to separate healing from what they saw as magical or supernatural qualities and laid the basis for modern science. He believed that disease resulted from natural, rather than supernatural, causes, and that these causes could be located through study and reason. However, like many of the healthcare systems that we now call nonconventional, Hippocrates believed in nature's healing ability and in a concept of health that involved wholeness and balance.

He taught physicians to study the patient, not just the illness. Each patient was a unique individual, who was an integral part of a greater environment that influenced his health and well-being in significant ways. A patient's environment, emotions and spiritual life all needed to be considered. In diagnosis, Hippocrates urged physicians to look at a wide range of factors, such as the patient's country and its

---

5 Hippocrates in The Heart of Healing, Turner Publishing, Inc., Atlanta, GA, 1993, p. 42

customs, diet, age, speech, behavior, sleep habits, dreams, even his silence and his thoughts.[6]

Likewise, Ayurvedic diagnosis is both detailed and comprehensive. It considers everything from the quality of the patient's physical constitution and mental perspective, to the nature of his speech; from his birthplace to his exercise regime.

Through thousands of years, Ayurveda has maintained the basic knowledge of health as wholeness. Maharishi has revived many of the lost dimensions of Ayurveda and given an understanding of wholeness which encompasses the entire universe, the totality of Natural Law. As you will see, the highest understanding of health and wholeness embraces not only a state of inner fulfillment and balance but also the harmonious integration and interaction of the individual with the entire cosmos. We need this universally comprehensive paradigm offered by Maharishi Vedic Medicine to treat and prevent complex conditions like arthritis effectively.

---

[6] The Institute of Noetic Sciences with William Poole, The Heart of Healing, Turner Publishing, Inc., Atlanta, GA, 1993, p. 49

Chapter Two

Arthritis: Living in the Kingdom of Aches and Pains

In this chapter we'll explore the nature of several of the most prevalent forms of arthritis from the perspective of allopathic medicine. We will see that a great variety of symptoms can arise with these conditions and that their prognosis can have unpredictable aspects. As a result, these diseases have presented medical science with enormous challenges in their search for comprehensive cures and clear causes, even with the help of advanced technology.

Arthritis

Arthritis means "inflamed joint." ("Arthros" means "joint" and "it is" means "inflammation.") The term "arthritis" covers a group of about 100 conditions, which involve inflammation in the joints and pain or discomfort in the connective tissue throughout the body. Inflammation is something that occurs normally whenever the body repairs damaged tissues. Damaged cells effuse a variety of substances, some of which attract white blood cells to the wounded area. The white blood cells clear damaged tissue while healthy replacement cells grow in. This work increases blood flow to the area which makes extra oxygen and nutrients available to support the healing activity. The increased blood flow produces warmth and redness; when fluid collects, swelling occurs. Pain arises when substances called prostaglandins[7] cause nerves in the damaged area to become extremely sensitive.

Inflammation is obviously a normal and essential process in tissue repair. However, if the tissue damage continues or if the inflammation itself causes damage, complications can arise. This is just what happens in many types of arthritis.

Approximately seventy-five million people, or about one in three Americans, have at least some pain in their bones or joints. For most of these people, the pain is minimal and short-lived. However, for some twenty million people the pain is stronger and sustained. Many of these people need medical help to do their jobs and maintain normal life. They feel pain whenever they move or walk or use their hands. About three million people have severe pain and other symptoms from arthritis even with medication and additional forms of treatment.[8]

Each year, United States surgeons perform 300,000 hip replacements, 300,000 lower back operations and 300,000 knee replacements, largely due to osteoarthritis. It's predicted that as many as ninety percent of Americans will get osteoarthritis at some point in their lives. Approximately two out of three people age thirty-five and older already have it.[9] However, this means that osteoarthritis is not inevitable: Ten percent of the population does not experience any joint degeneration. As you will see, MVM offers the knowledge

---

[7] When some part of your body is traumatizede.g., you sprain an ankle or fall harda long nerve cell which has connections to both your spinal cord and the affected area releases a chemical called substance P into your spinal cord. Substance P is essentially a molecule which activates pain signals. Substance P triggers the release of glutamate, a neurotransmitter, which in turn triggers the discharge of a chemical member of the prostaglandin family. This prostaglandin cues a spinal neuron linked with the brain to transmit the message that a painful event has taken place.

[8] Tiger, Steven, Understanding Disease-Arthritis, Simon & Schuster, New York, 1986, p. 8

[9] Bucci, L. op.cit., pp. 8-9.

of how to prevent as well as how to cure arthritis.

Our Brilliantly-Engineered Joints

Let's take a closer look at the beautifully engineered structure we call joints, which have now become a trouble spot for so many people. Human beings have 206 joints, or places where two or more bones come together. Joints allow bones to move and protect them from injury when they are in motion. Joint ends are covered by pads of cartilage, a tough spongy substance that acts much like a car bumper and keeps the bones from grinding against each other when they move. The joints are enclosed by a capsule that fits closely around the bones on each side. These capsules are constructed of tough fibers, including the thick strands we call ligaments. The fibers keep the joint together, while muscles surrounding the capsule and joint add support.

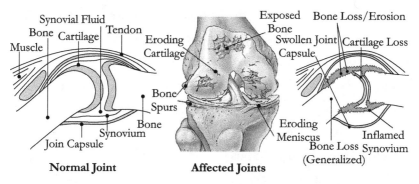

A thick solution, called synovial fluid fills the space inside the capsule and helps cushion the bones and lubricate the joints so that the bones can rotate without friction. Synovial fluid is produced by a membrane called the synovium, which lines the interior of the joint capsule. A small sac called a bursa is found near the joint but exterior to the capsule. It rests between the muscles and tendons and allows them to move over each other smoothly.

Rheumatoid Arthritis

Each part of the joint is essential for smooth functioning. Each of the many different forms of arthritis involves damage to one or more of the joint's components. Let's look at rheumatoid arthritis (RA), for example. Three times as many women as men suffer from RA. Mysteriously, the disease often improves or disappears when a woman gets pregnant, only to return six weeks after delivery. A number of infections seem to trigger RA, as do cold weather, stress and trauma, and it is inflammatory, not degenerative. This means that age and/or heavy exercise are not necessarily contributing factors.

In rheumatoid arthritis, the immune system's natural healing response goes awry. In addition to the natural inflammation process, the immune system produces antibodies to help get rid of any foreign substances, from a splinter to a virus. In rheumatoid arthritis, the body creates autoantibodies that attack the joints continuously and cause redness and swelling in the synovium, which lines and lubricates them. Fluid and pus flow into the encapsulated joint space as the body continues to try and rid itself of a foreign body. However, in the case of RA, no one seems to know what the foreign body is.
Chronic inflammation gradually results in significant damage to many joints, muscles and tendons and the consequence is pain and

limitations on activity. The small joints in the hands and feet are the ones most commonly effected, especially the knuckles and toes. However, RA can invade any joint, particularly those in the hands, wrists, elbows, feet, ankles, hips and knees. Secondary effects can include osteoarthritis and destruction of cartilage, bone and related ligaments; stiffness, fatigue, weight and appetite loss, aching muscles and a low grade fever.

Science has not yet located a definitive cause, though research began as early as 1858. A genetic or inherited tendency appears to be involved, which means that prevention measures can play a role in inhibiting its onset or severity. Other researchers believe that viral or bacterial infections and emotional stress are causative factors.

RA is unpredictable in terms of the frequency of its occurrences and the manifestation of its symptoms. For instance, some people only have one or two joints affected, while for others, the disease is widespread. Some patients experience red, painless nodules on the skin, and almost ninety percent have an antibody called the rheumatoid factor or titer in their blood. Ten percent of patients have a spontaneous remission in six months to two years of the start of RA,[10] while others experience ongoing debility for the rest of their lives, or alternate periods of normal health with occasional flare-ups. Because of these variations, and because it often begins gradually and with subtle symptoms, RA can be challenging to diagnose, especially in its early stages. As you will see, Maharishi Ayurvedic diagnostic techniques can be extremely useful in pinpointing the

---

10 Long, James W., M.D., The Essential Guide to Chronic Illness, Harper Collins Publishers, Inc., New York, 1997, p. 372

onset of RA. This is critical because the earlier that RA can be diagnosed and treated, the more effective the results will be.

At this time, allopathic medicine has no cure. This is not surprising since the cause is not fully comprehended and the disease takes on so many different appearances. Disease management usually needs to be individualized. Certain drugs are used to control inflammation and relieve pain (especially aspirin in large doses and NSAIDs-nonsteroidal anti-inflammatory drugs), and others are used to modify the actual progress of the disease and potentially produce a remission. Patient responses to drugs vary greatly and a certain amount of experimentation is often needed to determine the right medication for each patient. The range of side-effects can include anemia, kidney and liver damage, diarrhea, headaches, memory loss and confusion, sleeplessness, depression, nausea, ulcers, gastritis, high blood pressure, etc. Some drug reactions are severe, even life-threatening, but the average medication trial period lasts about two weeks and many doctors believe that the damage from dangerous responses is generally reversible when the medications are stopped.

Appropriate exercise is extremely important. Diet, nutritional supplements, massage, physical therapy, emotional counseling, techniques for joint protection and stress management are all increasingly recognized as useful in dealing with RA.

Osteoarthritis: Losing Our Natural Shock-Absorbers

If American life continues in its present pattern, nearly ninety percent of us will get some degree of osteoarthritis (OA) at some point in our lives, especially after age sixty. Quite a few people do not even know that they have this condition, as they have no pain or other obvious symptoms. Many physicians consider some degree of OA to be an inevitable part of the aging process. However, for a significant number of people, OA can be painful and debilitating.

OA results when cartilage, the spongy shock-absorber that covers our joint ends, deteriorates. When the cushioning between the bones is injured or starts to disappear, bones rub against bones. Stiffness and varying degrees of pain and loss of motion result. Eventually, bone grating against bone can produce osteophytes or spursuneven outgrowths on the bone-which can also grind against each other. Spinal spurs can also squeeze nerves and cause severe pain. The damage usually occurs gradually, over a number of years, and consequently OA is considered a degenerative disease.

Episodes of pain and stiffness might occur at intervals of months or even years. OA usually shows up in three places: the fingers, the spine and the weight-bearing joints: hips, knees and feet. While RA is an inflammatory disease that will attack many joints and other parts of the body, OA symptoms frequently show up in just one place. However, even when only one joint is affected, there are repercussions in other parts of the body. Muscles around or at a distance from the joint may tighten to avoid pain or protect the diseased joint. Healthy joints may start working abnormally hard to make up for weakness in the arthritic joint.

The primary cause for OA is unknown. Though OA is strongly associated with aging, the degenerative process can also be caused or speeded up by injuries, or by years of repetitive motion, or even by poor alignment. Its symptoms may appear early or late in life, simply because cartilage wears out for different people at different ages. Recent research has isolated a genetic defect that influences the development of osteoarthritis in the hands. Some researchers believe that damage to cartilage and/or its rebuilding are related to metabolic processes and that cartilage can be repaired through nutritional means and dietary changes.

As with other forms of arthritis, neither a definitive cause nor cure is available. Doctors seek to reduce pain and limit disabling effects. Various forms of pain medications are usually recommended, including NSAIDs (aspirin, Advil, Naprosyn) and acetaminophen (Tylenol-type drugs), but they all have side effects. Yes! Even the seemingly innocent aspirin can be dangerous. Aspirin inhibits the enzyme that makes prostaglandins.[11] Prostaglandin molecules either benefit or destroy; they either reduce pain and inflammation or create it. Aspirins (and other types of NSAIDs) inhibit both the good and bad kinds of prostaglandins. The high doses of aspirin recommended for arthritis can produce anything from queasiness to stomach ulcers to kidney damage.

---

11 Prostaglandins are important lipid-soluble molecules produced by almost every cell in the body. They are produced locally and serve as messengers. They exist only for seconds to minutes and strongly affect local function in such areas as inflammatory responses, blood pressure regulation and blood clotting.

NSAIDs in general tend to accumulate in the body and destroy prostaglandins. They can damage the stomach, liver, kidneys, immune and nervous systems, skin and bone marrow. Most significantly, certain NSAIDs can make the disease worse, while they prevent pain. These NSAIDs actually promote cartilage deterioration and prevent its repair.[12]

Moist heat therapy, corticosteroid injections, topical analgesics, weight control and exercise especially swimming-are all useful to either decrease pain or help maintain muscle strength and general mobility. When all other treatments have failed and a joint is virtually destroyed, joint replacement surgery is an option. More than three million Americans now have artificial joints and the surgery usually saved them from being crippled or wheelchair-bound.

So many people suffer from painful arthritis and cannot tolerate drugs that it is one of the major areas in which the population has sought nonconventional treatments. These include anti-inflammatory herbs, dietary nutrients that help repair cartilage (e.g., glucosamine and chondroitin sulfates) and combat free radicals; massage and other forms of muscle relaxation; acupuncture and special diets. Many of these therapies provide non-toxic approaches to combating symptoms, slowing down the progress of the disease and promoting better general health, but a complete cure remains elusive.

---

12 Bucci, L., op. cit., pp. 174-175

Fibromyalgia: Pain All Over

Fibromyalgia affects about five million Americans, eighty to ninety percent of whom are women between the ages of thirty-five and sixty. It is not a form of arthritis, though it is frequently misdiagnosed as such. It can disturb everyday functioning as much as RA and is actually more common.[13] In the past, fibromyalgia was often misunderstood, and allopathic physicians thought that complaints about symptoms were mostly psychosomatic. It was seen as a largely psychological disorder related to high susceptibility to stress or depression. Consequently, patients with significant pain were given the impression that their symptoms had no physical basis.

Today, stress is seen both as a cause and result of FMS (fibromyalgia syndrome), but in 1987, the American Medical Association recognized FMS as a genuine physiological disorder and major source of disability. It was officially diagnosed in 1993 for the World Health Organization as "a painful but not articular (not present in joints) condition, predominantly involving muscles, and as the most common cause of chronic, widespread musculoskeletal pain."[14] However, perhaps due to its complexity, many doctors still dismiss it or fail to differentiate it clearly from other conditions with chronic pain. Though the pattern of fibromyalgia's symptoms are fairly consistent, they are so broad that some doctors continue to feel that FMS may actually be a group of different diseases with similar

---

[13] Fransen, J., and Russell, I.J., op.cit., p. 3. Devin, M.D. and Copeland, Mary Ellen, M.S., M.A., Fibromyalgia & Chronic Myofascial
[14] Starlanyl, Pain Syndrome, A Survival Manual, New Harbinger Publications, Inc., Oakland, CA, 1996, pp. 8-9.

symptoms that cannot be distinguished.[15]

Currently, fibromyalgia is understood to be a disease that involves chronic diffuse pain in the muscles and surrounding structures. Certain characteristic points are particularly tender when palpated. Other symptoms can include fatigue, poor sleep, headaches, numbness and tingling, sensitivity to weather and temperature changes, sensitivity to stress and physical activity, anxiety and depression, morning stiffness, irritable bowel syndrome, joint pain, subjective swelling (a feeling of swelling when none is there) and difficulties with memory and concentration.

The function of neurotransmitters is negatively impacted and this in turn affects all functions which depend on muscle coordination and communication. In addition, FMS increases sensitivity in the nerve endings so that normal sensory input is interpreted as pain. Consequently, the body may frequently produce a "fight or flight" response, which, when inappropriate, results in a buildup of further muscle tension and anxiety.

The roots of FMS are unclear. Allopathic medicine notes potential causes as depression, physical or emotional trauma and CNS, the defect in neurotransmitters that leads to a distorted perception of pain. One study points to inheritance as a factor. The 1989 research indicated that nearly half of the children of an FMS parent are likely to contract the condition.[16]

Once again, medical science is faced with a complicated and

---
15 Fransen, J. and Russell, I.J., op. cit., p. 14.
16 Starlanyl, D. and Copeland, M.E., op.cit., p. 12.

unpredictable disease which is difficult to diagnose and heal. The course of FMS can vary from day to day. Flare-ups do not occur in any regular rhythm and conditions can change suddenly. FMS is largely treated with medications that address its symptoms: anti-inflammatory drugs for pain, sleep medication, muscle relaxants and anti-depressants. Due to the unpredictability of the disease's prognosis, the medications need regular monitoring by a physician. Most of them have side-effects, ranging from nausea, diarrhea and dizziness, to headaches, constipation, heart palpitations, sexual dysfunction and dependence.

The symptoms and their psychological fallout have also been relieved by massage, physical therapy and exercise, psychiatric care, various relaxation techniques and acupuncture. Though any patient in pain must be grateful for anything that brings relief, the process of maintaining freedom from pain is time-consuming, complex and costly, and allopathic medicine does not currently hold out any immediate hope for a cure.

Lupus

Systemic lupus, like rheumatoid arthritis, involves malfunctioning in the immune system. Lupus patients generate an unusually large number of abnormal antibodies that attack healthy tissue instead of battling foreign substances. It's as if the body becomes allergic to itself. Antibodies are protein molecules which the body produces to destroy foreign invaders. The immune system's B cells produce antibodies in response to the presence of foreign substances (antigens[17]) in order to eradicate them. In the case of lupus, the immune system, for no obvious reason, mistakes the body's own cells and tissues for foreign invaders and tries to kill them as it would a foreign material.

The antibody attacks often produce inflammation in the body's connective and vascular tissue. Since connective tissue is found in every organ and system, the tissue damage is not limited to joints and their surrounding area. Lupus involves the destruction of organs and tissues throughout the body-skin, heart, circulatory system, etc.

Science currently identifies three types of lupus:
(1) *Systemic lupus* can affect any and all physiological systems and its cause is unknown.
(2) *Discoid lupus* affects the skin and its cause is unknown. It can be a symptom of systemic lupus, but it usually occurs by itself.
(3) *Drug-induced lupus* is caused by taking in certain chemicals, including medicines. The three medicines which most commonly trigger lupus are Pronestyl (used to treat heart arrhythmias); Apresoline (used to treat high blood presssure); and INH, or isoniazid (used to treat tuberculosis). Genetics plays a role in susceptibility to drug-induced lupus, but is not the exclusive cause.[18]

Lupus affects about half a million people in the U.S., with 16,000 new cases being identified each year. Women have a much higher occurrence: Ninety to ninety-five percent of lupus patients are

---

17 Antigens are defined as all substances that are either made by the body or come from outside the body which the immune system identifies as foreign, all substances which trigger an immune response.
18 Lahita, Robert G., M.D., and Phillips, Robert H., Ph.D., Lupus, Everything You Need to Know, Avery Publishing Group, Garden City Park, NY, 1998, pp. 14-17.

between the ages of thirteen and forty and female.[19] Its cause is undefined, however, researchers are looking at genetic factors, the environment and the presence of certain sex hormones as partial determinants.[20]

As with RA, lupus is difficult to detect, because the symptoms and their expression vary so much. Its most common indicators include rashes, lesions or ulcers on the skin; chest pain and difficulty breathing; swelling, redness and pain in the joints; stomach pain and nausea; kidney dysfunction; weakness, fatigue, low-grade fevers and general achiness. It can take up to eight years to conclusively diagnose lupus, though any patient with both joint pain and a multi-system disease might be a candidate.

Lupus is not actually a form of arthritis, but over ninety percent of lupus patients experience arthritic conditions and arthritis can be an indicator of lupus. All the joints can be touched, but it most commonly strikes the fingers, wrists, elbows, shoulders, knees and feet. The early stages of lupus usually do not affect the hips and spine.

In lupus, the joint lining becomes inflamed when white cells in the joint area secrete inflammatory chemicals as part of the body's immune response. Fluid leakage from the blood vessels also occurs and the joints swell and become red-hot. Due to lupus, the soft tissue surrounding the joints, such as tendons and ligaments is destroyed but no bone erosion or joint destruction occurs. This is one of the main ways that it differs from OA and RA.

---

19 Eileen
20 Ibid. Radziunas, Lupus: My Search for a Diagnosis, Hunter House Inc., Claremont, CA, 1989, p. 103, p. 104.

Here again, physicians confront a complex condition whose cause remains a mystery. One book on lupus states: "Lupus patients all share similar symptoms, based on inflammatory processes. Fever, weakness, aches, and pains are all common aspects of this unique disease. We do not know how to treat these various symptom complexes. In essence, it is the symptoms that are being treated and not the real disease, since the actual cause is unknown."[21]

Without a clear picture of the cause and prognosis of lupus, present levels of treatment remain partial and only address relief from pain and other debilitating features. Doctors usually prescribe high-dose steroids or NSAIDs, which are associated with a depressing list of side-effects.

Gout: How Can a Toe Hurt So Much?

As a child I connected gout with rich, grumpy lords in English fairytales. In contemporary reality, more than one million Americans suffer from this disease and about ninety percent of them are men over the age of forty. Many gout patients are overweight and about a quarter of them have it in their family histories.[22] Gout involves chronic and intense inflammation in the joints. It occurs when high levels of uric acid in the bloodstream accumulate and form needle-like sodium monourale crystals, which get deposited in the joint fluid. Gout is extremely painful and most commonly strikes the big toe, but is sometimes found in other small joints as well-ankles, knees, wrists, elbows and fingers.

---

[21] Lahita and Phillips, op. cit., p. 23. Alan, D.C., Ph.D., and Goodman, Herbert D., M.D., Ph.D., Treating Arthritis, Carpal Tunnel Syndrome, and Joint Conditions, The Philip Lief Group, Inc., New York, NY, 1997, p. 108.
[22] Pressman,

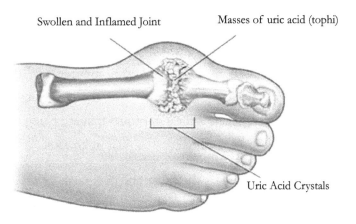

Swollen and Inflamed Joint
Masses of uric acid (tophi)
Uric Acid Crystals

The model for gout patients is an over-forty, overweight, successful man, whose life includes a significant amount of personal and professional aggravation. Frequently his diet will include a lot of alcohol and meat, both of which raise serum uric acid. High blood pressure and a low fitness level are also common characteristics.

Episodes of gout appear suddenly and can produce crippling pain. White blood cells assault the uric acid crystals and their struggle generates more crystals, which in turn attract more white blood cells. The result is inflammation and throbbing pain. For some, the attack comes only once in a lifetime, but for about half the patients, the attacks will increase in frequency and intensity. Preventive measures can play an important role. The first attack can serve as a wake-up call to make lifestyle changes. These may include diets which avoid or decrease uric acid and eliminate obesity, as well as stress management programs. Doctors also use ongoing medication to control uric acid levels in the blood. No permanent cure is available.

Immediate treatment usually focuses, of necessity, on pain relief. Anti-inflammatory medications are frequently recommended. Colchicine, widely used since about 1850, can relieve pain within forty-eight hours, but it may also produce nausea, vomiting, stomach cramps and diarrhea. A number of less-toxic NSAIDs are also prescribed, as are steroids, or even strong analgesics such as codeine if the pain cannot be reduced in any other way.

Ankylosing Spondylitis: The Stiff Spine

Ankylosing Spondylitis (AS) is arthritis of the spine and it affects about two million people in the United Sates. It strikes more men than women and usually starts in the twenties or thirties. It often runs in families and disease victims share a common genetic marker-the white blood cell group HL-B27. However, the presence of this gene does not make the disease inevitable. In fact, it is estimated that ninety-five percent of those with this marker never suffer from AS. A highly stressful event or an intestinal infection from one or more unknown bacteria may play a role in triggering AS.

In AS, when inflammation in the spinal joints subsides, a healing process occurs in which the bone grows out from both sides of the joint and eventually completely surrounds it. The joint can then no longer move and the resulting stiffness is called ankylosis. The early symptoms of AS resemble many other forms of back pain and it may go undetected for a long time. This is unfortunate because early identification and treatment are important to prevent the spread of inflammation and the development of deformities.

AS manifests quite differently in different people and its symptoms may come and go. It usually decreases in severity over time, but the lumbar spine stiffens and the upper back and neck may also harden. The inflammation initially produces stiffness and pain, but after awhile, a bony ridge grows between the parts and the whole area hardens and loses flexibility. AS therefore does not cause bone degeneration, but rather fuses the bones together. This process stops motion but also stops pain, as pain arises when the joints move.

With AS, doctors try to slow down the progress of the disease and minimize the symptoms. They have no cure and do not fully understand the causea situation which is probably starting to sound familiar. Typical treatments include, as usual, pain-relief (anti-inflammatory) medication, along with surgery for joint replacement when necessary. Physical therapy and exercise (especially swimming) to keep joint muscles strong and flexible; relaxation techniques to loosen muscles and enhance breathing; and maintaining good posture and normal weight all seem to slow down the effects of AS.

Repetitive Motion and Disease: Carpal Tunnel Syndrome

As more and more people hold jobs which require repetitive actions-from typing on a computer to working on assembly line-we are faced with a wave of related conditions, based on cumulative injury. Carpal tunnel syndrome, whose name is associated with the eight carpal bones in the wrist, is one of the most widespread and painful. Along with a ligament, the carpals form a tunnel-like framework that acts as a corridor for the tendons that control the movement of our fingers, and for the median nerve, which relays sensations and controls some movements of the thumb and several fingers. The painful condition called carpal tunnel syndrome arises when tendons swell and press on the median nerve. The median nerve can also be compressed by a cyst on a tendon, a tumor or inflammation from conditions like RA.

The tendons may swell due to forceful or repetitive movements or prolonged bending of the wrist involved in certain kinds of work or recreation. House painters, carpenters and violinists have been victims for years. Even sleeping on your hands can produce carpal tunnel syndrome. However, this disease was relatively unknown among the general population before we became glued to our computers. In the past ten years, the number of reported cases has actually tripled due to computer use, but also due to the spread of automated, specialized work that requires people to perform a few simple motions several thousand or more times per day every day. Unfortunately, repetitive injuries often produce a lot of secondary damage. Though hands and wrists suffer the most, the entire arm as well as upper back, neck and shoulder can suffer as we unconsciously try to compensate for the wrist pain. The pain might migrate from one spot to another from day to day.

Numbness and tingling are usually the first symptoms to appear. Later, victims may lose nerve sensation, which in turn leads to loss of hand coordination and strength. Disease victims might lose the ability to hold things, or to perform simple tasks like tying a shoe lace or opening a jar. They might also be unable to distinguish hot from cold with their hands, or find it difficult just to open and close them. Pain is a definite feature, some times localized, sometimes spread over a wide area, sometimes severe.

Early treatment of this disease can lead to a complete recovery, while ignoring the symptoms over a long period could lead to permanent damage. Hence the ability to diagnose early and correctly is extremely important. In the early stages, carpal tunnel syndrome may disappear completely simply by stopping the damaging activity. If this is not enough, splints are also used effectively. NSAIDs are used to bring down pain and inflammation. However, the potential side effects have to be watched, especially in patients over forty. Cortisone steroid injections also successfully reduce pain, but repeated injections into the same tendon can rupture it. Surgery is recommended when the situation is severe enough to produce nerve damage. Hydrotherapy, acupuncture and various forms of physical and movement therapy have been found to relax the injured area, relieve pain and increase flexibility and strength.

Had Enough?

Even though, we have only described a few of the most widespread forms of arthritis and joint conditions, perhaps at this point you are thinking that you have read enough. Uniformly, the causes of these conditions remain unknown. The disease symptoms are depressing to consider, and the most common treatment regimens involve drugs with some serious and scary side effects. Most people with these diseases are faced with unfortunate trade-offs simply to decrease their pain, as well as lifestyle considerations that not only consume large amounts of time but also dominate thoughts and feelings and that is just to slow the disease process down. Allopathy offers no cures at this time and none are promised for the immediate future. The only progress seems to be in creating less toxic and damaging pain-relief medications. The numbers of people affected are overwhelming. No wonder we are looking for solutions beyond the current offerings of conventional medicine.

It is interesting to consider that some of the heath care systems which we call alternative or nonconventional have actually been used for thousands of years, while allopathic medicine is only about three hundred years old. Moreover, eighty percent of the population of the world uses these ancient systems. Though all the latest knowledge and technology provided by modern science is available to Americans, and we spend more than trillions of dollars each year to use it, we are by no means the world's healthiest population. In fact, we are number forty-three on the international list. Perhaps it's time to combine the wisdom of East and West, old and new, and share the medical mainstream with a system of knowledge that has been helping people for many generations. As you will see in the next chapters, by taking its own objective techniques to their limits, Western medical science is in fact gradually approaching the same holistic understanding of the basis of health which Ayurveda has maintained over the centuries.

Chapter Three

The Miracle of Human Life

Miracles do not happen in contradiction of nature, but in contradiction of what we know about nature.[23]

Saint Augustine (A.D. 354-430)

Anyone who contemplates any single aspect of the human physiology-from the tiniest cell replete with DNA, to the ingenious composition of a joint or the efficiency and complexity of the immune system-has to be awed by the incredible engineering in each individual element of the human physiology. If we also look at the ways in which all the billions of parts work together, largely without conscious effort on our part, can we possibly see the human system in the same way that Descartes did-as a fantastic machine that runs by fixed rules, unrelated to any coordinating intelligence?

Even the simplest observation of every day activity-the ability to walk or cook or get out of bed in the morning-demonstrates the intimacy between mind and body. The slightest intention of the mind mobilizes a myriad of physiological responses to help us accomplish the thousands of movements that we take for granted in daily life. To describe all the physiological processes involved just in turning a doorknob would take pages and pages. It would probably take an advanced computer a week to track the activities of all the neurons, cells and systems needed for this simple gesture. Yet the mind/body

---

[23] The Institute of Noetic Sciences, The Heart of Healing, Turner Publishing, Inc., Atlanta, GA, 1993, p. 14.

instantly calculates and produces what is needed for both easy and highly complicated tasks every second of every day. Surely some magnificent intelligence must orchestrate all this.

Intelligence is something difficult to measure. It is so agile, dynamic and mutable that it cannot easily be studied through medicine's objective means. However, recent discoveries, particularly by endocrinologists, have provided a new sense of the nature of biological intelligence. Western medical science may in fact be leading us back to an understanding of the intimacy of mind and body and of health as wholeness that we lost 300 years ago. As they study the body's subtle chemical interactions, endocrinologists are finding that the mind guides every physiological process, and that what we understand as mind is found throughout the body, not just localized in the brain. Intelligence is pervasive and guides the activity and responses of every cell.

Intelligence Is Everywhere

Dr. Candace Pert, former chief of the brain biochemistry section at the National Institute of Mental Health, is a pioneer in the fascinating study of neuropeptides and information-carrying molecules. Scientists initially identified fifty or sixty neuropeptides-strands of amino acids, the building block of proteins-in the hypothalamus, the part of the brain that deals with emotions. These peptides along with other information molecules and their cellular receptors appear to be the biochemical correlates of emotions. They have now been found all over the brain and body, connecting every major system.

Neuropeptides serve as a kind of chemical interface between the mind and body, as they translate impulses of intelligence or emotion into physiological events. Acting as messengers, they travel around the body and link up with specific receptors found on nearly all our cells. Each of the millions of cells in the body has numerous receptor sites attached to it, which function much like satellite dishes, constantly adapting to receive the attracted messenger molecules. The linking process between information molecules and receptors is very specific, just like a lock and key. The connection triggers the receptor and a flood of responses in cells, tissues, organ, etc.

Based on her research, Dr. Pert observed that ". . . your brain is extremely well integrated with the rest of your body at a molecular level, so much so that the term mobile brain is an apt description of the psychosomatic network through which intelligent information travels from one system to another. . . Every second a massive information exchange is occurring in your body."[24] This picture of the body as an information network moves us ever further away from a mechanistic view of a body divorced from mind.

Our Dazzling Nervous System

Our brain cells or neurons communicate across gaps called synapses. Slender, branch-like threads called dendrites are found at the end of each neuron and these synapses separate the dendrites. We each have billions of these neurons and each one can sprout anywhere from dozens to hundreds of dendrites- an estimated 100 million million of

---

24 Pert, Candace B., Ph.D., Molecules of Emotion, Simon & Schuster, New York, NY, 1993, pp. 188-9.

them. This means that the potential number of combinations of signals leaping across the synapses in the nervous system is greater than the number of atoms in the known universe. Millions of signals interact instantaneously everysecond. For instance, to start your car this morning, your brain took only a few milliseconds to arrange the movement of millions of signals. Our nervous systems are amazing computers, designed to constantly handle immense numbers of bytes of information.

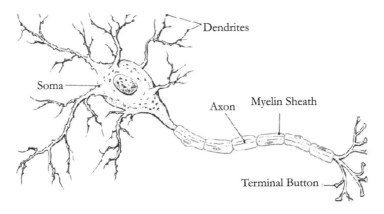

Many people still see the nervous system as a kind of super-efficient telephone system in which information is passed in a linear fashion down the axons or trunks of the neurons. However, we now know that information is passed via chemicals-neurotransmitters-not electrical impulses. These molecules are not found just in the brain and nervous system, but everywhere in the body-in the immune system, intestines, stomach, heart, bones, joints. This tells us that the brain is not the only source of the messages. Intelligence flows everywhere inside us via chemical messengers and receptors.

Neurotransmitters affect the function of every cell and circulate wherever thoughts want to travel. Each thought is a feat of brain chemistry which generates a surge of reactions throughout the body. We do not yet understand how this flood of biochemicals flows into patterns that parallel the mind's myriad functions, but Western science is beginning to detect the apparatus for the mind's projection into the body.

All of the body's biochemicals-enzymes, hormones, neurotransmitters, etc.-seem to know exactly which receptors they fit into. As we observe them, molecules appear to select the correct site, going straight to where they are needed, as if directed by a radar system attuned to the brain. In addition, we can release a multitude of biochemicals simultaneously and each one is coordinated with reference to the whole. To make things even more interesting, a neuron does not simply catch an impulse from the cell next door and transmit it as is to the next neuron. The neuron can change the message: It can transform the chemical it received. We have seen that the receptor sites on the ends of nerve cells are constantly adjusting to receive different types of messages. The broadcast station on the other side of a synapse is just as versatile.

DNA: Our Central Intelligence Agency

Every cell in our bodies comes from one double strand of DNA, created at the time of conception. That first molecule contains the blueprint for all that we do and become. DNA's expressions are immensely varied and specialized, but every cell in our bodies contains the totality of our DNA's possibilities. Neurotransmitters are just one of DNA's products. All of our protein is built from chains of twenty amino acids; when organized into longer strands, they are called peptides. Neuropeptides have their own distinct pattern, which makes them different from the body's other peptide chains, but they are all produced under the direction of DNA.

Encoded in the DNA in every cell is all the information necessary to create and maintain our lives. However, physically speaking, even DNA is composed of the same, basic chemical building blocks as the communicator molecules which it assembles and directs-strings of sugar, amines and other simple compounds. What directs all that massive organizing power? Is there an underlying intelligence?

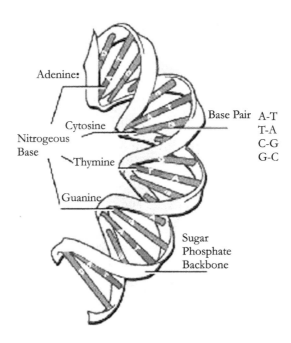

DNA's information is primarily fixed; it is the most stable chemical in the body. Now we have also identified more fluid counterparts of intelligence-neurotransmitters and other messenger molecules and their supremely versatile receptors, through which the mind can project itself everywhere and anywhere in the body. Every cell in the body can "think" and feel, because every cell has highly adaptive receptors for information molecules.

The discovery of information or messenger molecules has expanded our comprehension of physiological intelligence, but we still cannot explain why one messenger molecule vs. Another gets created in any particular moment. Each cell may have a great number of instructions that it can dispatch and receive, but it activates only a small fraction at any given time. Why do particular neuropeptides and neurotransmitters emerge and where do they come from? What produces daydreaming? What allows us to catch our balance just in time or step on the brakes at just the right moment?

The system of synapses and neurotransmitters provides a chemical channel through which our brains can talk to our bodies. The mind, which is non-physical, has found a way to work in intimate partnership with communicator molecules. The collaboration is profound. The mind essentially depends on these neurotransmitters to operate within the body, but it is not these chemicals.

Is there a guiding and coordinating intelligence, an organizing power for this immensely complex yet precise flow of physiological events?

Is there a way to verify its existence directly, not just through its apparent effects? Its influence seems to be present everywhere in the mind/body, not just the brain and nervous system. As Dr. Pert observes: "With information added to the process, we see that there is an intelligence running things. It's not a matter of energy acting on matter to create behavior, but of intelligence in the form of information running all the systems and creating behavior." [25]

If this vastly creative, management system, this powerful pervasive intelligence, functions perfectly and is fully available, then every cell and every system ought to operate perfectly and at its full potential. The ancient Ayurvedic system has always recognized this underlying intelligence. Accessing and aligning with that intelligence is in fact the key to health.

---

25 Pert, C., Ibid, p. 185.

Chapter Four

What Is Maharishi Vedic Medicine?

When the total intelligence of Natural Law Veda is lively in the individual physiology, there is perfect synchrony between the functioning of every individual cell and the holistic functioning of the body as a whole, and between individual intelligence and Cosmic intelligence. With this complete integration, all thought and action are spontaneously in harmony with Natural Law and the individual enjoys perfect health.

-Maharishi Mahesh Yogi[26]

When Carolyn first came to see me, she suffered from a host of uncomfortable symptoms: headaches, chronic fatigue, muscle soreness and joint pain, sinus pain, and digestive problems. In addition, she was overweight. "I just never feel good anymore," she confided. She was a thirty- two-year-old surgical nurse and her job was demanding, requiring a lot of concentration. Her most recent symptom had been failing concentration and short-term memory loss.

She had been diagnosed with both arthritis and fibromyalgia. Her doctors had prescribed anti-inflammatory drugs but they upset her stomach and made her feel nauseous. Medication for her sinuses produced diarrhea and disturbed sleep. As the final disaster, she suffered from PMS mood swings and migraine headaches both before and during her periods. Understandably, Carolyn was starting

---

[26] Maharishi Mahesh Yogi, Maharishi Forum of Natural Law and National Law for Doctors, Age of Enlightenment Publications, India, 1995, p. 11.

to feel desperate. "I"m too young to have this many problems," she told me. "I just want to feel good again." After one month of using Maharishi Vedic Medicine (MVM), she had made impressive progress. She reported: "I feel better in many ways. I'm sleeping better and I lost eight pounds since my first visit. My sinus problems have improved, my digestion is better and I don't have stomach pain or nausea." Though Carolyn's joint pain and muscle pain remained, her PMS discomfort had also decreased.

The second month of MVM produced even more breakthroughs. "I have fewer headaches. I seem to have a lot more energy and cope with my work better. The muscle soreness is still there, but it's improving. When two more months passed, both Carolyn's energy level and digestion were in good shape. She had suffered no headaches in the previous six weeks, and her muscle and joint pain had continued to decrease. When Carolyn had been following MVM's recommendations for a total of nine months, everything felt better. Her joint pain was minimal and her muscle pain was significantly improved.

At this point, I put Carolyn on an MVM health maintenance routine. I see her every three months and she continues to do well. As you might expect, she's extremely happy that she found Maharishi Vedic Medicine.

Comprehensive Healing

Carolyn's history is just one among many success stories. As I look at the tired, sometimes despairing, faces of people like Carolyn, I feel greatly relieved that they have at last found their way to my office door. I know that MVM is going to turn their lives around. How is it that this system of medicine can relieve widespread symptoms in such a short period of time?

Though it is certainly necessary to alleviate acute symptoms such as pain, trying to heal one symptom at a time is like trying to help a sick tree by painting each leaf green. It does not get to the root of the problem. Any healing that takes place is piecemeal. Ayurvedic healthcare is based on alignment with the most fundamental level of life, a field of pure intelligence or consciousness, the essential nature of every atom and every cell. Using Ayurveda's principles and treatment regimens creates balance and healing at the root of life. As a result, the healing is comprehensive and complete.

Ayurveda is part of a system of knowledge called Veda, which is available to us in the Sanskrit language. Veda means "knowledge" and ayu means "life." Ayurveda, then, roughly translates as "complete knowledge of life." The idea of complete knowledge incorporates not only an understanding of human life, but of the life of the entire universe. As you will see, a number of Ayurvedic therapies recognize our deep interconnectedness with the rest of the universe and work to bring us into harmony with the laws and rhythms of the cosmos.

The Managing Intelligence of the Universe

The Sanskrit sounds of the Vedic texts and the order of their appearance embody the process of the creation and evolution of the universe. The complex but orderly flow of events, that results in our concrete world, begins from undifferentiated wholeness, or pure awareness. This unified wholeness contains within itself the potential for all that exists, in much the same way that a seed contains the total potential for a tree. Many quantum physicists today theorize that the force and matter fields which structure our creation emerge from one unified field. The unified field of pure, unlimited potential toward which their research points is the Veda.

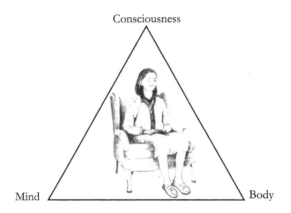

Veda is pure consciousness, pure intelligence. It is the fundamental nature of the manifest world, and it contains the total potential of all the natural laws and forces that create and maintain it. The total potential of natural law governing the universe exists like an eternal blueprint for creation in the field of the Veda, the unmanifest basis of all life.

In the sequence and flow of its syllables and words, and in the structure of its presentation, the Vedic literature expresses the process of creation from underlying wholeness. The laws of nature emerge from the unified state of natural law-which in Sanskrit is called samhita-in an orderly and predictable way. However, the wholeness at the basis of creation remains present in each and every step of diversification. Pure consciousness, pure intelligence, permeates every part of creation. As Maharishi Mahesh Yogi explains:

The unified field progresses sequentially. There is the sequential progression of the unified field into the specificities of life, the space-time boundaries of life. It is always a sequential development. Sequential development means that the whole tree is found in the seed. The whole tree is found in the first stage of sprouting of the seed, and in the second stage of sprouting, and in the third stage of sprouting. As the tree grows, the total tree is contained at every level. This is Vedic Literature. It unfolds as natural law unfolds, from its total basis in the unified field to its specific expressions. Like that, sequentially developing, the whole infinite diversity of the universe is created and maintained and kept self-referral[27]

For all the knowledge that science has given us, our universe remains a vast and mysterious place. If you traveled in a spaceship going ten miles per second, it would take you three-and-a-half months to reach the sun and seventy thousand years to reach the nearest star, Alpha Centauri. The Andromeda galaxy, which has almost twice as many stars as our own Milky Way, is about twelve quintillion (that's eighteen zeros!) miles from us. At best guess, scientists estimate the existence of one hundred billion galaxies, each one of which contains hundreds of thousands of millions of stars. It is difficult

---

[27] Dillbeck, Michael. C.,"Self-Interacting Dynamics of Consciousness," in Modern Science and Vedic Science, Maharishi University of Management, Fairfield, IA, 1988, pp. 250-251.

even to conceive of the immensity of the universe, the types of life forms which might exist and the number of cosmic events occurring each moment. Even the best science fiction can't do justice to the possibilities.

Closer to home, we know that the universe's amazing level of structure and organization is displayed not only in its immensity but also in the tiniest cells in every living form. All this emerges from consciousness, the Veda, the total potential of Natural Law—and all this is orchestrated by the infinite intelligence and organizing power of this all-pervasive unified field of pure being. Pure consciousness is the managing intelligence of the universe.

Veda 101

Though we do not expect you to grasp all this in one quick reading, we do want you to have at least a glimpse of the big picture. If you can understand even a little about the nature of consciousness and the Veda, you will have a sense of why the Ayurvedic health care system is so deep and complete in its effects. On the basis of this broad understanding, we hope you will be able to apply some of the practical recommendations that we give in later chapters for addressing arthritis with greater discernment and satisfaction.

First, how does abstract field of pure awareness become matter? It does so in a precisely ordered process, which the Veda expresses in the quality and order of its sounds. The transformations of consciousness that give rise to matter are expressed as sound or vibration, and the forms that emerge are inherent in the sounds. All the concrete, material forms and phenomena in creation are expressions of the Vedic sounds, which are vibratory impulses of consciousness. Similarly quantum physics describes all particles of matter as modes of excitation of underlying fields. Because pure consciousness and pure intelligence are one and the same, the condition for consciousness to know itself, to be aware of its own nature, is present at the basis of creation. This self-referral, self-knowing, nature of consciousness is the origin of its creativity. In the mechanics of knowing itself, pure consciousness gives rise to three basic components of experience: knower (rishi), process of knowing (devata) and object of knowing or observing (chhandas). The interaction of these three elements produces the specific and precise patterns of vibration of the Veda.

Though they have been written down, these sounds are not the creation or speculation of individual minds. Rather they are "heard" or cognized by individuals as they clearly experienced pure awareness and its eternal dynamic within themselves.

The Veda is a sequential embodiment of or commentary on the process by which the unified field of natural law manifests as the rich, unlimited diversity of creation. Each stage of emergence of the Veda and the Vedic literature is a further description of the process of creation, or an elaboration of the unfolding of the totality of natural law that exists in seed form in the unified field. This is not a process that develops over time, but one which is complete and continuous through what we know as time.

The sounds of the Veda, then, are the vibratory patterns of matter as we know it. All the forms which matter takes are the concrete, precipitated expressions of these sounds. Certain aspects of the Veda express the transmutations in consciousness which precipitate into matter. Another aspect of the Vedic literature, Upaveda (subordinate Veda), describes the dynamics of transformation in the world of matter that gets created-the dynamics which enhance the reawakening of consciousness in matter, or of wholeness in the vast diversity of creation. Ayurveda is the main branch of the Upavedic texts. Maharishi describes Ayurveda for us as follows:

In the sequential growth, consciousness becomes matter. Then what we find is that the field of Veda as consciousness is over and the field of Ayur-Veda has come up to deal with matter.

The Upaveda, or subordinate Vedas, present the knowledge of how to enliven the Veda as a living reality on the level of one's own existence. The Upavedas ... handle the most expressed value of natural law in which consciousness has assumed the quality of matter, providing the principles and techniques through which matter can be reenlivened with the full value of consciousness.[28]

The Primary Cause of Disease

Maharishi Vedic Medicine both prevents and alleviates disease by restoring the connection of every part of the body-every atom, cell and organ-with the pure intelligence at its source. For health, the behavior of each and every part must be fully governed by the underlying wholeness, the unmanifest blueprint for perfect form and function. In fact, MVM defines the primary cause of all sickness as

---

28 Dillbeck, M. C., op. cit., p. 258.

pragyaparadh, "the mistake of the intellect." When we are only aware of diversity-the content of our thoughts, the objects of our senses-and we have lost our experience of wholeness, we open ourselves to the possibility for either psychological or physical illness.

When we "forget" the underlying unity, when we conceptually[29] disconnect from it, some part of us will start to function in an abnormal or disorderly way, both within itself and in terms of its coordination with the whole mind/body. Remember that the entire creation, including our bodies, consists of increasingly complex and elaborate expressions of pure consciousness. When our experience of consciousness is limited or obscured because we are totally absorbed in material experience, a kind of shadow is created in the mind/body. We are cut off from the full value of Nature's managing intelligence and things can go awry. It's like a factory with a director who's distracted from his job, or a director with only a partial knowledge of the purpose and production needs of the factory. Some things get manufactured incorrectly; others not at all. Parts produced on one side of the factory don't fit or work with those from another area. If no comprehensive managing force is instituted, many mistakes are made and even chaos could result.

According to Ayurvedic physician and researcher Dr. Hari Sharma, disease is the equivalent of "an invasion of disorder," due to clouded access to pure consciousness. "The expressions of the Body's healing intelligence are expressions of the internal dynamics of wholeness, restoring the coordinated, harmonious functioning of

---

[29] According to the Vedic understanding of life, we can never actually disconnect from our own true nature. However, we can lose our conscious access to or awareness of it.

the human physiology. Therefore, if disease is present, our first concern should not be so much with the diseased parts, as with how wholeness can be reenlivened."[30]

Universal Patterns of Orderliness

The focus of science has been to discover the underlying design in nature's functioning, to locate laws, or regular patterns and relationships in the vast multiplicity of creation. In searching for these laws, we are implying our belief in an underlying orderliness. Our universe could have been totally devoid of such patterns of orderliness, a chaotic system in which no stable states of matter could develop. However, physicists today are aware that the self-organization of matter and energy into increasingly complex and elegant forms is possible only because of specific conditions.

Einstein once stated his belief that God doesn't play dice with the universe. As our observations of the universe on both a microscopic and macroscopic scale become more accurate and sophisticated, we are, in fact, able to see the tremendous precision with which the universe is created and orchestrated, whether we look at immense galaxies or tiny atoms. In fact, the microscopic and macroscopic levels of creation are intimately related. Stars are produced by interactions at the subatomic level of matter. Carbon, an element critical to life forms, is the result of thermodynamic reactions in the core of stars.

---

[30] Sharma, Hari, M.D., Awakening Nature's Healing Inelligence, Lotus Press, Twin Lakes, WI, 1997, p. 68.

The more science discovers about the ingenious design of our human organism, the more we must assume an underlying managing intelligence. Physicist Paul Davies writes:

The main reason why the origin of life is such a puzzle is because the spontaneous appearance of such elaborate and organized complexity seems so improbable. . . . the level of complexity of a real organism is enormously greater than that of mere amino acids . . . The complexity needed involves certain specific chemical forms and reactions: a random complex network of reactions is unlikely to yield life."[31]

The direction of science has been to locate not only regular patterns or laws of nature's functioning but also deeper, more all-encompassing laws and forces. In recent years, physics concluded that all known physical interactions were governed by four fundamental forces: gravity, the strong and weak nuclear forces and electromagnetism. They then saw that this could be further reduced: The grand unification theory united electromagnetism and the strong and weak nuclear forces. Many physicists today are confident that the model for a completely unified field theory, which joins all four major force fields and their associated matter, is inevitable. This picture of the basis of creation would allow us to see every force and matter field as a vibrational expression of the underlying unified field. In confirming the existence a unified field, physics will have rediscovered the ancient Vedic paradigm, which describes the material creation as an expression of an underlying field of pure intelligence.

---

31 Davies, P., op.cit., P.27

MVM's paths to reestablishing unity with Nature's infinite intelligence leads to a quality of health based on the full potential of life and complete harmony with natural law.

. . .The self-referral state of consciousness is the one element in nature on the ground of which the infinite variety of creation is continuously emerging, growing, and dissolving. The whole field of change comes from the field of non-change, from this self- referral, immortal state of consciousness. The interaction of the different intellectually conceived components of this unified, self-referral state of consciousness is that all- powerful activity at the most elementary level of nature. That activity is responsible for the innumerable varieties of life in the world, the innumerable streams of intelligence in creation. If this state of consciousness, or this state of nature's activity, could be brought on the level of daily life, then life would naturally be as orderly and as full of all possibilities as is the nature of this self-referral state of consciousness.[32]

Ayurveda contains many paths back to connectedness with Nature's infinite intelligence and organizing power. MVM has taken on the job of making these paths available in the simplest and most effective forms of treatment. To understand and fully use these treatments, we need to have a clear picture of the major components of Ayurvedic physiology.

---

32 Dillbeck, M.C., op. cit., pp. 273-274.

Chapter Five

The Components of Balance: Template for a Pain-Free Life

When the total intelligence of Natural Law-Veda-is lively in the individual physiology, there is perfect synchrony between the functioning of every individual cell and the holistic functioning of the body as a whole, and between individual intelligence and Cosmic intelligence. With this complete integration, all thought and action are spontaneously in harmony with Natural Law and the individual enjoys perfect health.[33]

Maharishi Mahesh Yogi

We know now that the basis for Ayurvedic healing is reenlivening wholeness in every part of the mind/body. When we work with that understanding, even complex, longstanding conditions can be helped quickly. I remember, for instance treating a bright, alert woman of eighty-one, named Alice. She had numerous problems, including high blood pressure and peripheral vascular disease, which produced numbness and tingling in her lower extremities, forearms and hands. For the previous ten years, she had had lower back pain and joint pain, especially in the knees and had been told that she had osteoarthritis. She loved walking but both the peripheral vascular disease and arthritis were making this difficult.

Her doctors had painted a hopeless picture with regard to the vascular disease and had recommended surgery to prevent worsening symptoms. She was on high blood pressure medication

---

[33] Maharishi Mahesh Yogi, Maharishi Forum of Natural Law and National Law for Doctors, Age of Enlightenment Publications, India, 1995, p. 11.

and her initial blood pressure was 172/94. All my prescriptions-which included herbs, dietary changes and a self-oil massage-aimed at eliminating deep constitutional imbalances which shadowed Alice's physiological connection to Nature's pure intelligence. The positive results were both comprehensive and quick to arise.

When I saw Alice again after one month, her blood pressure had come down to 113/78, and she reported experiencing less tingling and numbness in her lower extremities and less lower back and joint pain. She was able to walk more and I was also able to prescribe some gentle exercise MVM yoga postures-to increase flexibility and circulation. Her blood pressure medicine had been cut in half.

After two months on her MVM regimen, she was able to eliminate her blood pressure medication. Her back pain and a lot of the numbness in her lower legs had disappeared. Alice continued to check in with me every eight weeks, and after just over a year of treatment, both her arthritis symptoms and the numbness in her feet were gone, and only minimal tingling remained in her fingers.

I continue to see Alice every two to three months. She is maintaining a dietary and lifestyle routine that keeps her arthritis in check and she experiences very little pain or numbness. She was surprised at how much could be accomplished without surgery. She is not only free of pain but is enjoying an active life.

Ayurvedic Anatomy

We'll now explore the basics of what I'll call Ayurvedic anatomy, so that you can understand the Ayurvedic approach to healing more completely. As we explained in the last chapter, the material world emerges from consciousness in a definite sequence. In addition, we could say that the underlying field of pure intelligence is infinitely aware. Because it is infinitely aware, its must be aware of something. In the state of undifferentiated wholeness, there is nothing for consciousness to be aware of except itself. That is why it is called a self-referral state of consciousness. In knowing or being aware if itself, consciousness takes on a kind of unmanifest infrastructure: the three-fold values of rishi, devata and chhandas (knower, process of knowing and object of knowledge). It does so without losing its unified state, because this three-fold infrastructure is virtual. The three-in-one structure of consciousness ultimately gives rise to all the diversity of creation, as consciousness in a sense fully explores its own nature, its unlimited potential.

As Dr. Sharma describes it:

After the initial division of one into three, consciousness starts experiencing all the possible modes of knowing itself. In a stepwise progression, the original three interact an infinite number of times, assuming infinite degrees of shadings and complexities. All subjects and objects in the universe, along with the relationships between them, emerge as the passing configurations of unbounded pure consciousness knowing itself in its infinite range of possibilities... Each mode of consciousness knowing itself has a specific vibrational quality associated with it. All the expressions of creation-material or nonmaterial-are ultimately nothing but these specific vibrational frequencies."[34]

---

34 Sharma, Hari, M.D., op. cit., pp. 106-7

The Vedic texts call the wholeness which permeates creation Atma, or Self. The first "quality" to arise from Atma is the ego, the sense of "I-ness," the most refined value of life. The ego is the "small" self, the inner experiencer. The ego feels, understands and thinks. The ego is the I in "I have" or "I know."

The aspect of the ego that thinks becomes mind, or manas. The faculty of the ego which understands, discriminates and decides becomes intellect. Here, the understanding of mind covers all mental activity and structure. The mind receives all the impulses of sensory information from our every day experience. It considers possibilities and relationships and also provides memory. The intellect evaluates what comes in. Is it good or bad? Do we keep it and use it or reject it?

The Three Mental Qualities

Mind has central significance in MVM and is found throughout the body. In Ayurveda, three specific qualities called gunas color the functioning of the mind, rather like colored lenses on eyeglasses. The mind's dominant quality colors our general outlook and our interpretation of sensory input. This in turn determines our body's responses to experience and is therefore critical to health.

As we learned earlier, even from the perspective of contemporary endocrinology, our minds and emotions are not localized, but are found everywhere in the body. Our thoughts and feelings are constantly being translated into physiological events. The balance of the three gunas or qualities in manas (the mind) influence whether those events support health or disease.

Let's look at some examples of how the mind leads the body. People who feel they are too busy to get sick usually have above average health. People who feel that they are always running out of time often die younger than those who feel they have ample time. The leading cause of death in the United States is heart disease, but the prognosis of the disease is very personal. People whose arteries are 85% blocked have run marathons while others with clear arteries have died of heart attacks. Similarly, the rhythm of rheumatic flare-ups can vary widely from one patient to the next. Individuals with multiple personalities have actually been known to display different diseases when they switch personalities. One personality may manifest full-blown diabetes, while another is free of diabetes but suffering from food allergies.

The three gunas-rajas, sattwa and tamas-can be understood as phases of activity. Rajas is the force of activation and organization, while sattwa and tamas uphold the direction of movement. Sattwa maintains and tamas ends, completes or slows things down. All three are present not only in the mind but also in every process in creation, no matter how small or large. The creative aspect of sattwa helps take every process into its next stage. Through sattwa, things begin, life is born. Tamas checks or retards each process in order to maintain whatever has already been produced, so that it can provide the foundation for the next stage.[35]

In the mind, sattwa results in the desire to know, as well as the ability

---

[35] Maharishi Mahesh Yogi, On the Bhagavad-Gita, A New Translation and Commentary Chapters 1-6, Penguin Books, Baltimore, MD, 1969, p. 120

to create, think and imagine. It gets expressed as curiosity, happiness and inspiration. Rajas generates activity and gets expressed in the ability to organize, achieve and execute. Tamas supplies the mind with the ability to complete whatever was started and carried out by sattwa and rajas.

Suppose you wanted to start a new business. Sattwa provides the inspiration and imagination for the new business. It supports the vision of its structure and purpose and perhaps the content of the mission statement and initial business plan. However, it remains just an idea until rajas helps you turn the plan into a physical reality—build the infrastructure, find the financing, hire the employees, etc. Tamas helps complete the building phase so that you can actually move into production. Otherwise, you might spend forever in the start-up process.

Or, perhaps you want to improve your health. This desire comes from sattwa. The efforts you make, such as doing research on the internet or reading this book or seeing an MVM physician, come from rajas. Tamas, however, might lead you to give up, feel like it is too hard to change or forget why you were inspired in the first place.

Because atma (the Self) is fundamentally creative, the natural balance of the gunas in the mind is characterized by the predominance of sattwa, with rajas and tamas having less influence. It is extremely important for health that we maintain this natural balance. When the mind loses this balance, we find the potential for disease. The sattwic mind maintains its full relationship with pure intelligence. It chooses things that support growth and happiness, that uphold and sustain life. You will see how important this is when we discuss the relationship between lifestyle, diet and both the prevention and cure of arthritis.

When patients with a sattwic nature meet with a doctor, they are clear about their symptoms and cooperative. They follow the doctor's treatment plan. They usually want a larger perspective on their illness and why they fell ill. They take responsibility for their health and usually don't want to rely on doctors or medication.

When tamas increases in the mind, we feel dull, lethargic, or even depressed. We tend to make damaging lifestyle choices and mistakes in many areas of life and find it difficult to accomplish anything. Our connection with our body's managing intelligence is cloudy at best. If we visit a doctor, we probably won't follow through on his or her recommendations.

The rajasic temperament is pressured and overstimulated. When rajas predominates, we lose all sense of inner peace and don't know how to stop, even at night. Our minds keep racing even when our bodies are exhausted. Patients with strong rajas might exaggerate their symptoms when they visit a doctor, or express irritation or desperation. They are prone to dependency on physicians and drugs and may seek one doctor after another.

A rajasic mind tends to choose experiences that overload and damage the senses, such as loud music or terrifying movies. Tamas dulls the receptive capacity of the senses, which may then send distorted or incomplete messages to the mind about the body or the environment. However, when the mind is sattwic, the information from our senses is accurately received and transmitted, and our ability to discriminate is finely tuned. We choose experiences that protect, nourish and strengthen every part of our lives and our connection to the environment.

The Five Elements

After the subjective stages of life-mind, intellect, ego-have unfolded, we find the first appearance of the objective world. The finest level of matter arises as five basic forces or elements, which have both subtle and gross values. In their subtlest expression, they are known as tanmatras. The tanmatras are the essences, or the intelligent blueprint, of the objects of the five senses. They exist at the subtlest level of creation, at the borderline between consciousness and matter. The Vedic description of the tanmatras at the finest level of material existence corresponds with the picture of the emergence of creation provided by quantum physics. Modern physics has located five major spin types, which give rise to all the elementary particles. According to physicist, Dr. John Hagelin, the properties of these spin types resemble those of the Tanmatras.

The Five Mahabhutas

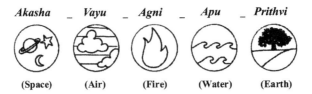

Five mahabhutas arise from the tanmatras as their slightly more concrete expression. They are the basic building blocks of the entire physical creation, including, of course, the human body. They emerge in order from subtlest to most concrete.

Most of us will have no trouble identifying the last four elements, but "space" may be new or unfamiliar. Very simply, it is the element that surrounds us all the time. It is what we move through when we walk or run. When we stand at the top of a mountain and look out over miles of vista, it is part of the freedom and expansion that we see and feel. Akasha allows us to have knowledge of things within our range of perception. We usually think of air as the element that surrounds us, but space is finer than air and precedes it in the order of creation. It is a kind of matrix in which the other elements can manifest.

We call *vayu* "air," but it is much more than that. It is a form of intelligence or natural law that originates and gives direction to all movement and change in the universe, from the rotation of electrons around a nucleus to the immense swirling of galaxies. Vayu (movement) must take place in akasha (space). Light and heat, associated with agni, are generated from the friction and pressure in movement.

Agni is responsible for all conversion and transformation processes. The light and heat of the sun result from powerful nuclear reactions in its core. The sun or agni is the primary source of the heat necessary for all conversion events in our bodies and on our planet, whether it is the metabolism of food or the production of carbohydrates in plants.

Apu or *Jala* enables cohesion and liquidity. It supports the ability of any substance to move or change shape without falling apart or losing its integrity. Dry earth, for instance, crumbles in your hand, while moist earth holds together. Jala is the main constituent of all life forms and water is its main expression. As water, it is responsible for increasing the size of organic forms. It is jala that lubricates and protects joints so that the bones can move over one another.

Prithvi provides substance and structure. The influence of prithvi is found in anything that has a shape, whether it's a cell or a solar system. We associate it with earth, and it helps determine the form and structure of every plant, tree and mountain, as well as every bone, muscle and organ. In our bodies, each of the elements is associated with a sense and sense organ. Our senses connect our inner subjective realm with material experience. Akasha is found in sound, the sense of hearing and the ears. Vayu is found in the sense of touch and the skin. Fire is connected to the eyes and the sense of sight, while water is found in the sense of taste and the tongue. Earth is related to the nose and the sense of smell.

Doshas: The Fundamentals of Balance

At the next stage of manifestation, the five mahabhutas merge into three basic mind/body operators or psycho-physiological principals called doshas: vata, pitta and kapha. Every cell in the body contains all three doshas, and the body needs all three to maintain life. Vata is the principle of movement and governs every motion in the body, from blood circulation, to the flow of impulses through the nervous system to the bending of a knee or finger. Pitta is the principle of heat and conducts all the body's heat-related and conversion processes, including metabolism, temperature and energy production. Kapha directs or is involved in creating and maintaining the body's physical structure-bones, fat, muscle, etc. as well as its fluid balance and lymph system. Its builds and holds cells together.

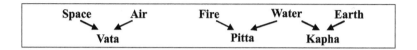

When I meet with arthritis patients, I find, of course, that many of them are suffering from similar symptoms. However, an arthritis ache in the hands or back can be a function of almost a hundred different forms of the disease. Though some people inherit the tendency toward arthritis, a tremendous array of other factors can encourage its development: stress, diet, too much or too little exercise and injuries and hormonal changes, to name a few. It is necessary to look much more deeply at what is going on in my patients physiologies and life circumstances before I can outline a therapeutic program for them.

The recommendations I make for treatment may be quite different from one patient to the next, even if on the surface they seem to be suffering from the same illness. In MVM, we treat the patient, not the disease, and one of the most significant pieces of information I have to understand patients is their doshic constitution, or prakriti. Each person is born with a personal, natural balance of the doshas. Some people have even amounts of all three (sama dosha), while others are dominated by one or two of the doshaskapha-vata or pitta-kapha, etc. This inborn, dynamic equilibrium of the doshas is each person's individualized pattern for health. Disturbance of that innate balance lays the groundwork for most mental and physical illness.

Through a variety of precise diagnostic techniques, some of which I will discuss later, I can detect both the natural balance of the doshas and any alteration of that state. The treatments prescribed by MVM largely aim to normalize or balance doshic activity in each individual, because the doshic constitution is each individual's blueprint for health.

The doshas pervade the subtlest level of creation. If you use your imagination, you can think of them as being so fine that they are on the borderline of physical reality where thought turns into matter. They are just material enough to be able to circulate throughout the body, to increase and decrease and accumulate in different cells and tissues. They are nature's operators, her agents of change and her functional intelligence. Though they are not visible, they have distinct qualities which we can observe throughout nature-and that physicians can observe in their patients. These are the qualities of the five mahabhutas (basic elements in Nature)

The Basic Qualities of the Doshas

Vata

mobile, light, quick, cold, changeable, rough, dry, subtle, leads the other doshas.

Pitta

slightly oily, hot, sharp, fluid, pungent, light, sour

Kapha

heavy, cold. soft, oily, sweet, steady, sticky, moist, slow, smooth, dull, dense

The Doshas in Detail

Since the doshas are an important part of Maharishi Vedic medicine, let's look at some of the simple ways we can identify them in our bodies. Vata dosha is cold and can lead to cold fingers, noses and feet and a dislike of cold, dry weather. Because it is dry, it can produce chapped, dry or cracked skin, or even psoriasis. This drying quality also plays a role in the development of arthritis, especially osteoarthritis. It is also responsible for the increased joint stiffness we feel as we age or even when the weather turns cold. Its roughness can make our hair feel coarse or our skin feel rough.

Vata's quickness can influence the mind both to learn fast and forget fast. It can also produce restlessness or impulsiveness, poor concentration, scattered thinking and the inability to relax. It generates alertness, creativity and a lively imagination. The quality of movement can yield either good or poor circulation, and it controls the efficiency of the nervous system and the process of elimination. Vata is light, subtle and penetrating and associated with acute pain.

Due to its mobility, vata leads the other doshas. In fact, sometimes vata is called the king of the doshas, because it moves all three of them and all their products throughout the body. Its mobile quality can spread imbalance, disease and its byproducts, and it plays a role in conditions with symptoms which spread throughout the body, such as FMS or lupus. Vata also maintains the continuous, healthy, coordinated movement of the vast array of our physiological components: blood cells, nerve impulses, nutrients, waste matter, neurotransmitters, etc.

An individual with a vata-dominant constitution could have many of the following physical and psychological qualities:

A light, thin frame, difficult to gain weight; bones either very light or long and heavy; prominent joints, tendons and veins; cracking joints
Rough, dry skin; dark, dry, kinky hair
Teeth which are either very small or large, crooked and protruding
Small, dark, or dull eyes
Irregular appetite and energy level; irregular bursts of energy
Physically and mentally restless; moves and speaks quickly; tends to overexert and tire easily
Thrives on change; dislikes routine; maintains irregular lifestyle
Light, interrupted sleep; fear, running and flying in dreams
Learns quickly; forgets quickly
Tendency toward worry, anxiety and fear; excitable; frequent mood changes
Enthusiastic and imaginative

Pitta is associated with heat. It is involved in skin rashes, flushed skin and all inflammations including all forms of joint inflammation. It can generate either too much heat in the digestive tract, or a strong, efficient metabolism. It creates a good appetite and a dislike of hot weather. Pitta's sharpness leads to a quick, astute, highly focused mind, but also, potentially, to sharp speech. It can also generate high acidity in the stomach or elsewhere in the body, a cause of gout. Pitta's sour quality can result in bad breath, or bad-smelling excretions as well as sour body odors.

Pitta-dominant individuals can have many of the following attributes:

Medium build, strength and weight; relatively easy to maintain weight
Strong appetite, thirst and digestion. Eating late or skipping meals results in irritability or ravenous hunger.
Likes challenges but physical energy and stamina is moderate
Straight, fine hair that is red, blond or sandy; early grey; baldness and thinning hair
Sharp, penetrating eyes, medium in size; often green or grey; poor eyesight; eyes that redden easily; primarily visual response to life
Warm, soft, fair skin that burns easily; freckles and moles; prone to skin irritations, such as rashes, inflammations and acne
Strong intellect and sharp, precise speech; articulate; good public speakers; good memory; good concentration;
enterprising; excellent managers and leaders (except when sarcastic or abrasive); likes to be on time and productive
Can be irritable, hot-tempered, opinionated and argumentative, jealous (when imbalanced) or joyful, confident and courageous (when balanced)
Dislikes bright light, too much sun and hot weather
Particularly sensitive to impure food, toxic environments, alcohol, tobacco, and toxic emotions (anger, jealousy, hatred, etc.)
Sound sleep; dreams with anger, fire, war, violence

We find kapha dosha wherever the quality of heaviness shows up, for example, slow digestion, overweight, depression, sluggishness and lethargy. Kapha produces slow speech, movement and thinking and a slow, more methodical pace of learning, but a good long-term memory. Kapha is also associated with softness-soft skin and hair; large, soft eyes; an easygoing way of dealing with life. Kapha creates an influence of sweetness and stability. Kapha-dominant people have fewer mood changes, more compassion and forgiveness and less reactivity to life's challenges.

Kapha types are also characterized by:

Large, solid, powerful build, with lots of strength and endurance; wide hips and shoulders; curvaceous form
Slow, steady appetite, not much thirst; slow eater; gains weight easily and struggles to lose it; places a lot of
importance on food; responses dominated by taste and smell
Slow, graceful movement; tendency towards lethargy; needs demanding, regular exercise and stimulation in work and routine
Learns slowly, but good long-term memory; thorough; slow, deliberate speech
Dislikes cold, damp weather, that can cause depression
Long, deep sleep; water dreams; sexual dreams
Difficulty getting going in the morning
Compassionate, emotionally steady, forgiving, affectionate, self-contained; but can also procrastinate, become dull, depressed, lazy, stubborn, and attached to the past or the status quo

Each dosha has major and minor sites in the body, where it naturally dominates physiological activity.

Vata: Chief site is the large intestine. Secondary sites are the waist, thighs, bones, ears and skin.

Pitta: Chief site is the area around the navel. Secondary sites are the stomach, duodenum, small intestine, liver, spleen, pancreas, lymph, blood, sweat, eyes and skin.

Kapha: Chief site is the chest. Secondary sites are the throat, head, pancreas, joints, stomach, fat, tongue and nose.

Diagnosing doshic activity is quite detailed and precise because each dosha expresses itself through major subdivisions of its influence, which are called subdoshas.

The Five Subdoshas of Vata

1. Prana Vata
Meaning : Vital breath
Site: Head and brain, chest
Function : Breathing, sneezing first to move (including heart and respirator swallowing, belching throat, tongue, mouth, nose

Prana vata facilitates perception; enlivens the ability to think, reason and feel; creates clarity, alertness, exhilaration. It governs the rhythms of breathing and swallowing. Its movement is upward and connected to higher functions. Anxiety, insomnia, asthma, headaches, breathing problems and neurological disorders are all potential symptoms of imbalances in prana vata.

2. Udana Vata
Meaning : Moving upwards
Site: Navel, chest, throat
Function : Speech, singing; effort, creating energy, strength; Complexion

Udana vata controls speech, memory and the flow of thought. Its imbalances can result in fatigue, earaches, tonsillitis, sore throats and speech defects.

3. Samana Vata
Meaning : Moving easily
Site: The channels (srotas) that carry sweat, doshas and fluids Near agni (digestive fire)
Function : Fanning agni (digestive fire), supporting digestion

Samana vata promotes peristalsis and the movement of food and nutrients through the digestive tract. When imbalanced, digestion will be either too slow or too fast, which may result in gas, diarrhea, bloating or poor assimilation.

4. Apana Vata
Meaning : Moving downwards
Site: The colon and lower abdomen, testicles, penis, urinary Bladder, thighs, groin Rectum
Function : Elimination offeces, Complexion urine, semen and menstrual blood; delivery of the foetus

This subdosha moves downward and governs elimination, menstruation and sexual function. One of its locations, the large intestine, is vata's primary seat. When apana vata is out of balance, it can cause constipation, diarrhea, colitis, menstrual or intestinal cramps, lower back pain and sexual dysfunction.

5. Vyana Vata
Meaning : Moving in different directions; diffusely
Site: All over the body
Function : General body movements: extensions, contractions

Vyana vata is found everywhere in the body, via the skin and the nervous and circulatory systems. It controls blood pressure and heart rhythm, all facets of circulation and the sensation of touch. It also regulates sweating, yawning and blinking. Its imbalances can cause high or low blood pressure, problems with circulation and stress-related diseases.

The Five Subdoshas of Pitta

1. Pachaka Pitta
Meaning : To digest, cook, transform
Site: Duodenum, small intestine
Function : Digestion; maintaining the digestive fire

Pachaka pitta regulates the heat available for digestion and thus determines to a large extent the strength of digestion, It regulates the separation of nutrients from waste products. When aggravated, it can cause heartburn, stomach acid, ulcers and digestion that is either too fast or too slow.

2. Ranjaka Pitta
Meaning : To color
Site: Liver, spleen, duodenum
Function : Gives color to and forms the blood

Ranjaka pitta orchestrates the production of red blood cells, balances the blood chemistry and distributes nutrients via the blood. Environmental toxins ingested through food, air or water, as well as alcohol and tobacco, can derange ranjaka pitta. When imbalanced, it can cause anger, anemia, blood disorders and rashes.

3. Sadhaka Pitta
Meaning : To achieve, fulfill
Site: Heart
Function : Governs intelligence, desires, understanding, memory, ego, enthusiasm, energy; eliminates delusions

Sadhaka pitta governs the physical heart as well as the heart's feelings. It can produce joy and contentment or anger and sadness. It can give courage or the inability to face challenges and make decisions.

4. Alochaka Pitta
Meaning : To see completely
Site: Visual system, the eyes and visual cortex including
Function : Outer and inner vision

Alochaka pitta produces good or impaired vision. Emotions can often be seen in the eyes or affect their functioninge.g., going blind with anger or reflecting excitementand alochaka pitta links the eyes with emotions.

5. Brajaka Pitta
Meaning : To light or shine
Site: Skin
Function : Gives luster and color to the skin; regulates

Brajaka pitta can connect skin with our emotions, through blushing, for example. It can reflect hot emotions through red spots, rashes, acne and boils. When healthy, it provides a radiant, shiny, vital quality to the skin.

The Five Subdoshas of Kapha

1. Kledaka Kapha
Meaning : To moisten
Site: Stomach
Function : Moistening and initial digestion of food absorption through the Skin

Kledaka kapha is responsible for keeping the stomach lining moist and is important for digestion. When kapha is out of balance, it often shows up first in the stomach, creating slow or heavy digestion.

2. Avalambaka Kapha
Meaning : Double supporting
Site: Chest, heart, lower back
Function : Supports the heart and lumbar region

Avalambaka kapha provides strong muscles, protects the heart and keeps the chest, lungs and back strong. When imbalanced, conditions such as asthma, chest congestion and congestive heart failure can arise. Smoking has a particularly bad affect on this subdosha.

3. Bodhaka Kapha
Meaning : To obtain knowledge
Site: Tongue, throat
Function : Moistens the tongue, perceives taste, secretes mucous in the mouth

Bodhaka kapha governs taste, which is a primary factor in Ayurveda in both the determination of diet and medicines. Ayurveda describes six tastes and says all six must be available at each meal, both to balance the doshas and to feel satisfied. The taste buds can be desensitized when we repeatedly consume only a few of the tastes. When our taste buds lose their sharpness, other kapha problems can arise: obesity, allergies, congestion and diabetes.

4. Tarpaka Kapha
Meaning : To nourish and please
Site: Head
Function : Nourishes the mind, senses and motor Organs

Healthy tarpaka kapha is fluid and mobile. To protect the sense organs, it lubricates the nose, mouth and eyes. It also maintains the cerebrospinal fluid, critical for the central nervous system. When imbalanced, it becomes either congested or runny. Symptoms of imbalance include clogged sinuses, hay fever, sinus headaches and dull senses, especially smell.

5. Sleshaka Kapha
Meaning : To stick, bind, cohere
Site: Joints
Function : Lubricates the joints; provides binding and cohesion all over the Body

Most kapha imbalances show up in the chest area and spread upward into the head. The exception is imbalances involving sleshaka kapha, which lubricates every joint in the body. It is obviously a major player in many types of joint dysfunction.

Mary's Story

Now that you have this basic introduction to the nature and qualities of the doshas, you can understand how much this knowledge helped me to diagnose and treat a patient named Mary. When I first saw Mary, she was sixty years old and desperate. She was suffering from osteoarthritis in both her joints and spine. She also had a history of high blood pressure and sinus problems and her doctors had prescribed medicine to bring down her blood pressure. Mary reacted so severely to the medication that she had to be hospitalized. The doctors stopped the prescription, but discovered that she was borderline hypothyroid. Mary was given medicine for this, but reacted poorly to it; she felt flushed and dizzy. Her physicians stopped the first recommendation and prescribed another thyroid drug, but Mary couldn't tolerate that one either. While taking the prescribed medicines, Mary developed many uncomfortable symptoms, which continued even after she ceased taking the medicines. She had feelings of extreme fatigue, stomach pains, itchy skin, great thirst, burning feet and heat and redness in her face. By the time Mary came to my office, she was off all medications, including pain medication for arthritis, due to her intolerance. However, she still felt tremendous heat in her body. She was flushed and many parts of her body were covered with red patches. She felt hot to the touch. Her doctors couldn't understand her excessive heat and thirst. Her blood pressure was 144/92.

I found great imbalances in all three doshas, but pitta was most serious as I would have expected from all the heat she was experiencing. Rather than addressing each individual symptom-an almost impossible job-I prescribed a special diet and herbs to rebalance the doshas and reestablish health from the deepest physiological level. Mary noticed improvement even in the first few days of following this regimen.

When I saw Mary again after three months, her blood pressure had normalized and the excessive heat and thirst were gone. She had lost six pounds effortlessly and her sinus problems were minimal. Her thyroid function had grown more stable on its own and she was free of rashes and hot flashes, Her doctors were surprised at the speed, effectiveness and simplicity of the treatment. Mary's words to me reflected her relief. "Dr Reddy, there are so many patients like me who cannot tolerate the medicines and who react so adversely that it is life threatening. There is not much help out there. I'm so lucky I found you."

The Doshic Stages of Life

Ayurveda describes three major periods of life and each one is dominated by a different dosha. Kapha rules birth through puberty, as this is the body's major growth period. Kapha adds size and substance, and children continue to grow almost no matter what they eat. However, the quality of nourishment at this time is extremely important as it provides the building blocks for the adult body, piece by piece. The most common forms of illness in these early years are kaphic in nature: colds and sore throats, ear infections, respiratory problems, etc.

Pitta's influence increases in the mind/body from puberty to about middle age. The predominance of growth, of increases in size and mass, shifts to the development of reproductive potential, due to the transforming qualities of pitta. During puberty, the development in size and substance slows down and the body develops distinct sexual characteristics. Pitta-related symptoms, such as skin disorders, emotional swings and a bottomless appetite, can arise during this time. After puberty and into adulthood, pitta's fire gives us the courage, drive, energy and vision to achieve our ambitions and meet life's challenges. If pitta is too strong or too weak, digestive disturbances will increase.

In middle age, we experience a shift to vata dominance. Vata dosha brings the qualities of dryness, separation, motion and coolness to the fore. Our skin dries and wrinkles. Hair thins and grays, and we may lose weight, muscle tone and even height. We lose our tolerance for cold weather (which increases vata in the body) and joints stiffen.

Some tissues start to dehydrate and waste away and metabolism is disrupted. We may start to experience vata-based illnesses, such as insomnia, short-term memory loss, anxiety and a variety of neurological and degenerative diseases. Osteoarthritis, you may recall, is one disease commonly associated with the increased, vata-associated dryness that comes with advancing years.

During the kapha and pitta stages of life, we may not experience many uncomfortable disease symptoms, even if we have imbalances. However, once the vata phase starts, we are no longer able to avoid the symptoms. What was an occasional discomfort, a relatively soft signal from our bodies that all was not well, may now become a full blown disease, if we have not corrected the imbalance earlier. If toxins and wastes have built up in the body during the kapha and pitta periods, vata's quality of motion now concentrates the toxins in weak tissues. This disrupts tissue metabolism and deprives tissues of proper nutrition, resulting in serious illnesses. Diseases that manifest during the vata period are more difficult to treat because they are strengthened by an unchangeable natural cycle. This is why many doctors hope, at best, to manage arthritic symptoms that manifest in later years and do not expect a total cure. With arthritis, as with most other forms of illness, prevention and early intervention are therefore extremely important. As we progress through the book, we will discuss the tools and treatments provided by MVM to help catch and eliminate disease in its earliest stages. They will involve recommendations in three major areas: proper diet, treatment and behavior or lifestyle. Regular visits to a doctor trained in MVM can be a major preventive tool as we are trained to detect doshic imbalances at their very inception.

The Doshas are Everywhere

In Maharishi Vedic Medicine, an individual is never seen in isolation. To be healthy, we must maintain an harmonious alignment with both our immediate environment and the cosmos as a whole. We can actively participate in creating this alignment when we recognize that the same doshas that operate throughout our mind/body are at work throughout creation. Everything in and around us functions in cycles. Our minds and bodies are intimately linked to all the natural cycles—night and day, seasons, movements of the planets, etc. Our internal doshic equilibrium is directly affected by the doshic cycles in our immediate and distant environment. When we live in harmony with those cycles, it positively affects our inner balance and health. Let's look a little more closely at how this works

The Doshas and the Daily Cycle

Within a twenty-four hour cycle, different doshas predominate at different times of the day and night:

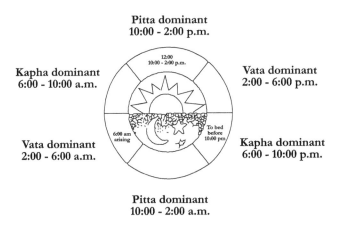

The Doshas and the Seasonal Cycle

Each season is dominated by one of the doshas. We are an intimate part of nature, so when a particular dosha is stronger in our outer environment, it also increases in our bodies, our inner environment. According to the Ayurvedic criteria, in North America, we have three seasons.

Spring (March-June) is dominated by the cool, moist influence of kapha. Everything begins to grow and take on size and substance. During this time, you might feel some heaviness and your digestion could slow down. Allergies, asthmas, colds, and sinus congestion become more common. If you suffer from rheumatoid arthritis or simple joint pain, symptoms may increase during kapha season.

Summer (July-October) is dominated by pitta's heat and transformational properties. Flowers bloom and fruits and vegetables emerge. The extra heat inside and outside may bring on headaches, rashes, irritability or excessive thirst. Heat-related conditions like gout or any joint inflammation may become more severe when pitta increases.

Winter (November-February) is dominated by the cold, dry, windy influence of vata. Your skin could become extra dry, and you might feel worried and anxious or have difficulty sleeping. Osteoarthritic symptoms such as joint pain and stiffness will frequently worsen in a cold, dry climate.

The Doshas and the Digestive Cycle

Each hour after eating is dominated by the particular dosha responsible for that stage of digestion. Kapha increases in the first hour after eating, pitta in the second hour and vata in the third. The next chapter will describe the digestive process in detail as it is critical both to creating health and the progress of disease.

Ayurvedic medicine is keenly aware of all these natural cycles and their importance to the quality of our daily lives and our health. The diets and behavioral routines prescribed by MVM physicians take into account not only the patient's individual constitution but also his or her geographical and seasonal environment. The routines recommended will help balance the seasonal doshic increase as well as any internal problems. The instructions for taking herbal compounds and other forms of treatment are related to the body's internal cycles. The body will make better use of certain herbs if we take them in the morning, or on a full stomach or an empty one, etc.

The Transcendental Meditation® (TM®) Technique

One of the most powerful and immediate ways to create inner balance, maintain sattwa in the mind and live in harmony with the environment is to practice the TM technique. I recommend it to my patients because it produces such comprehensive benefits with a relatively small time commitment: twenty minutes twice a day. Though it is essential to learn TM from a qualified instructor, once you learn, it becomes a potent, but absolutely easy and genuinely pleasant form of self-treatment. Students are always surprised at the total effortlessness of this practice and at how quickly they learn. In fact, it takes only a four-session course to master it.

Each time you practice the Transcendental Meditation program, your awareness expands to its infinite source in the field of pure consciousness. This helps reestablish that connectedness to the field of pure intelligence which Maharishi Vedic Medicine describes as the basis of health. At the same time, your body gains a profound state of rest-two or three times as deep as the rest in deep sleep. Rest is the fundamental condition for all healing. No one recovers from illness without extra rest, and some things, like broken bones and sprained ankles, heal just with rest. When the mind/body achieves this unusually deep rest during the TM practice, it immediately starts to throw off the stress and fatigue that you have been accumulating over a lifetime. I would like to emphasize that the TM technique is not a "stress-management" practice. It goes far beyond managing or coping, which I feel is a very limited expectation for life. It actually helps the mind/body permanently eliminate stress, and the shifts in health and behavior are large and surprising.

A tremendous amount of research-more than 600 studies-documents the benefits of this practice to every area of life. They include: increased intelligence; better memory; more energy, productivity and motivation; enhanced creativity; improved learning ability and academic performance; better overall health and immune function; reduced risk of heart disease; better mind-body coordination and athletic performance; slow-down of the ageing process; greater happiness, self-esteem and self-confidence; better relationships; and inner peace-to name a few!

As an MVM physician, I am particularly interested in having my patients become self-sufficient in their personal health care. This is a primary goal of Maharishi Vedic Medicine. In addition to the benefits defined by science, I notice that the patients who use the TM technique regularly, experience a host of automatic behavioral changes. As stress leaves the system, destructive Lifestyle habits such as smoking and poor diet often fall off. Even drug and alcohol abuse are positively affected. I often feel that if the TM technique were made available in the schools that our national drug problem would simply disappear. Studies done on students in the 1960s and 1970s showed that the vast majority spontaneously gave up using drugs simply as a result of their TM practice. Students (and adults) who use the TM technique are also far less likely ever to resort to drugs and alcohol, because their psychological health is so strong. They feel centered. They know who they are inside and they like who they know. Their intelligence, creativity and success levels are high. Life is an adventure, something to be treasured, and the impulse to escape or destroy life is just not there.

You may recall from Chapter Two that many forms of arthritis are either partially caused or complicated by stress and strong emotions. As inner stress levels are reduced through the TM practice, our emotions become more balanced, more positive, and our responses to environmental stress reflect that inner balance and sense of well-being. We begin to react appropriately to life's challenges, as opposed to over- or under-reacting. (Hyper-reactivity is one cause for intensification of FMS symptoms) To the degree that stress levels complicate our illness, the TM technique will provide relief. It will also help us deal with the fact of illness-and the accompanying pain and limitations-without becoming heavily overshadowed by our situation. The TM technique alone is probably not going to eliminate arthritic pain, but it can create the inner framework that allows us to be grateful for life, irrespective of disease.

When my patients make the TM technique part of their daily health routine, they tend to follow the whole treatment regimen more regularly and completely. They are motivated, even when goodhealth returns, to have a diet and lifestyle that maintains health and growth, so that future disease is prevented. The deep rest experienced during TM facilitates healing, while the transcending process promotes the reestablishment of the natural dominance of sattwa in the mind and reconnects you to the infinite organizing power of nature. You start to make better choices in all areas of life so that health can become a continuous reality. In the next chapter, it will be come clear just how important diet and lifestyle choices can be in the treatment (and prevention) of arthritis and many other diseases. simply disappear.

Chapter Six

Digestion: The Pivotal Process

He whose doshas are in balance, whose appetite is good, whose dhatus are functioning normally, whose malas are in balance, and whose body, mind and senses remain full of bliss, is called a healthy individual.[36]

Every patient that I see receives specific dietary recommendations which help eliminate accumulated toxins in the body and strengthen and balance the digestive process. June, for instance, was a fifty-five-year-old musician who came to see me several years ago. She reported that ever since receiving silicon breast implants, she had suffered from serious fatigue, digestive problems and aches and pains in all her joints and muscles, which gradually became persistent. Her doctors had given a diagnosis of fibromyositis and arthritis as well as chronic fatigue. They had prescribed anti-inflammatory medicines which had not helped much and had produced many side-effects, including heartburn, poor appetite, gas and bloating.

When she came to see me, she felt hopeless and helpless. Because the breast implants were a potential source of her problems, she had had them removed, but her symptoms had continued. I prescribed specific dietary changes to balance her doshas and reduce toxins. I also recommended a number of herbal formulas to correct imbalances in her digestion and help with constipation, sleep problems and both FMS and arthritis symptoms.

---
36 Sushrut, Surtrasthanam, 15:38.

Within a few weeks of starting her MVM regimen, her energy increased and she felt some relief from her aches and pains. Her digestion also started to improve. Over the next six months, her joint and muscle pain were significantly reduced. After one year, the pain related to arthritis and FMS were almost completely gone. The parallel improvements in June's digestion and joint and muscle pain were something that MVM would predict, because in Maharishi Vedic Medicine, digestion is a key player both in the healing and prevention of disease.

To understand the Ayurvedic picture of digestion, we have to look into the nature of agni. We often translate "agni" as "fire," but it has a more complex reality and a multitude of roles in our body. Agni is associated with the immense heat and light of the sun. It manifests the qualities of heat and thermogenesis throughout the universe, from the simple burning of wood into ashes to the powerful conversion processes taking place at the core of stars. In the digestive process, agni is called jatharagni. It manifests as our digestive fire, in our appetite and in the digestive secretions which break down and transform food into products that can be assimilated by cells and tissues.

As an element, agni has no clear form in our bodies; it cannot be located or identified through particular qualities. However, when it takes the form of pitta dosha, it becomes perceptible because it assumes the appearance of all five elements. For instance, when it materializes as one of the subdoshas of pittapachak pitta it displays the qualities of digestive secretions. As such, it can move and flow, is slightly oily, has a sour smell and taste and a yellow, green or reddish color.

Ayurveda describes thirteen forms or aspects of agni and each of these plays a role in changing food into blood, bone, tissues, etc. Jatharagni functions much like a cooking fire. It facilitates the first level of digestion in the gastro-intestinal tract, breaking down food into useable components. Jatharagni contains five bhutagnis that help process food composed of their corresponding elements. Apagni, for example, helps metabolize watery food, while prithivi agni helps process earth-dominant or heavier foods. Once food is sufficiently broken down, the digestive product, called aharasa, is absorbed into the circulatory system through the walls of the G-I tract and the process of building and nourishing the body's tissues begins.

During digestion in the gastro-intestinal tract, if one dosha predominates due to the nature of the food consumed, poor eating habits, or existing imbalances, the aharasa will carry that excess or aggravated dosha into the circulatory system and possibly to every tissue. Here lies the start of disease. For instance, putting excess vata into circulation could be the seed for any number of conditions, including most forms of arthritis and FMS. Excess pitta could lay the groundwork for gout. This kind of problem is not yet in itself a recognizable illness, but it lays the foundation for disease if not corrected.

The Seven Sequential Tissues

Once the aharasa is absorbed into circulation, another process begins. We call it metabolism and it is responsible for building all the body's tissues. In Ayurvedic physiology, the body is made up of seven tissues, or dhatus, which are built up in a fixed sequence. "Tissue," as we understand it does not encompass the complete meaning of the Ayurvedic dhatus. The dhatus are not always solid, nor do they always have a fixed form. Ayurveda defines dhatus as those substances and structures that the body retains and that are continuously rejuvenated and replenished. They are a natural part of the body's composition, and provide it with both physical mass and integrity. Each dhatu is associated with a specific form of agni (dhatu agni) which assists in the conversion of one tissue into the next. The work of each dhatu agni is highly specialized as it transforms one level of tissue into another. Each dhatu is essentially a metabolic refinement of the previous one. The order of tissue genesis and the corresponding dhatu agni are as follows:

Tissue	Dhatu Agni
Rasa (Plasma, chyle, the first product of digestion)	***Rasagni***
Rakta (Blood cells, erythrocytes, including hemoglobin)	***Raktagni***
Mamsa (Muscle)	***Mamsagni***
Meda (Fat)	***Medagni***
Asthi (Bone)	***Asthagni***
Majja (Bone marrow and central nervous system)	***Majjagni***
Shukra (Reproductive material)	***Shukragni***

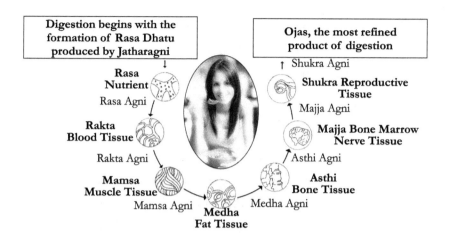

The work of the dhatu agnis and their corresponding tissues runs in sequence until all the tissues have been nourished and produced. This process of dhatu creation and conversion runs continuously in a cyclical order. The cycle from rasa to shukra can be immediate with some foods such as milk, or it might take six or even forty-two days.

The strength and health of each dhatu agni directly affects the health of its associated tissue. For instance, if mamsagni (muscle tissue agni) is low, muscles may not form properly and an individual might feel weak or experience muscle tissue degeneration. A disturbance in mamsa dhatu might also be a factor in fibromyalgia. Dysfunctional asthagni (bone tissue agni) could exacerbate certain forms of arthritis, while disruptions in medagni (fat tissue agni) could result in too much weight gain or loss.

The effectiveness of the dhatu agnis are dependent on the health of jatharagni, the digestive fire. When jatharagni is strong, the first tissue produced, rasadhatu, will be a clear, thin, odorless fluid which can permeate even the finest pores and cells of the body. Rasadhatu nourishes all the other dhatus, carrying essential nutrients to each tissue as it is transformed into the next one in the sequence.

If jatharagni becomes imbalanced or disturbed, food in the gastro-intestinal tract is inadequately or improperly broken down, and nutrient substances that are either unhealthy or unuseable are produced. If jatharagni is weak, the result is incompletely digested food that cannot be assimilated. If it is too strong, the food will be "burned" and its nutritional value partially destroyed. If jatharagni is unstable, digestion will probably generate a mixture of useful substances and undigested food.

A variety of factors can derange agni, including fasting, overeating, irregular eating habits, eating unhealthy food or eating before the previous meal is digested. Negative emotions-anger, worry, fear, etc. can also throw agni out of its natural state, as well as inadequate adaptation to geographical, climatic or seasonal changes.

Ama: Gumming Up the Works

When agni, and therefore digestion, is abnormal, ama, a sticky, toxic, sometimes- malodorous material gets created from the remains of poorly digested food. If one ultimate bad guy exists in the Ayurvedic paradigm, it is ama. As you will see, ama can seriously gum up the works and be a primary factor in almost every disease process, arthritis or otherwise. In fact, many of the recommendations we will give you in this book aim at reducing ama and preventing its formation. If agni is sufficiently disturbed, the digestive process generates a large amount of ama, which pollutes the digestive product, aharasa, the same way chemicals or algae pollute a clear mountain stream. This contaminated aharasa is absorbed into the circulatory system through the walls of the G-I tract where it in turn corrupts the rasadhatu. This refined nutrient fluid congeals; it becomes clouded and gooey and often develops a foul odor. Thick with impurities, it can no longer penetrate into the body's smallest pores and cells. In this adulterated form, rasadhatu cannot adequately nourish the other tissues. Unable to reach the tissue cells, it collects outside them and causes swelling. This is one of the primary causes of the swollen joints found in many forms of arthritis.

If the rasa dhatu is carrying both aggravated or excess doshas and ama into the circulatory system, we have one more building block for disease. For instance, if ama mixes with vata and it settles in the joints, we have the foundation for rheumatoid arthritis. If it also invades and settles in the muscle tissue, we have the basis for FMS. However, the first movement of ama and imbalanced doshas into the tissues usually causes only slight discomfort. Only when it has built up over a long period, do we have real disease. The first stages of imbalance are easily corrected and that is why in MVM we lay so much importance on early detection and prevention.

The Srotas: A System for Communicating and Getting Around

Ama can accumulate in and clog the body's transportation and communication system, called srotas. Srotas-defined as any space in the body-connect every cell, tissue and organ system. They vary widely in size and shape, and include large, visible channels, such as veins, arteries, lymph passages, tear ducts, the mouth and nose and millions of passageways that are too small to be seen. These tiny srotas are part of the dhatus. They are made of the same elements as the dhatu in which they reside, and are named after it. For example, the srotas that transport blood are called raktavaha srotas.

The srotas in each tissue carry the nutrient fluid to each cell and carry waste products away from them. They function with great precision. Each srota will only allow the specific nutrient that it is designed to carry to move through it, and the task of one type of srota cannot be done by another. The srotas in the bones, for example, only transport substances used to build or maintain bones.

When the srotas carry the nutrients to the tissue cells, the dhatu agni metabolizes the nutrients. (Remember that the dhatu agni is the tissue-specific digestive secretions that transform nutrients into tissue.) As the dhatu agni "digests" the nutrient material, three substances are created:

- Nutritional compounds which stay in the cells to sustain them and form new tissue.
- Nutrients which move out of the cells and are carried by rasa dhatu to feed the next tissue
- Waste products that are also transported through the srotas via rasa dhatu

The srotas thus support all areas of tissue metabolism by allowing the necessary movements and exchanges to take place. They also move the doshas throughout the body.

Srotas are classified into four major types:

- **Intake Srotas:** Passageways to move the breath (respiratory system); convey food (digestive system); move water and regulate water metabolism
- **Dhatu Srotas:** Passageways to carry plasma to blood and tissue (lymph and circulatory systems); circulate blood and hemoglobin; nourish bones, muscles and fat; feed bone marrow and nerve and brain cells (nervous system); transport semen and feed the male reproductive system

The Types of Srotas

Intake Srotas

1. Channels that transport breath, or prana: respiratory system (pranavaha srotas)
2. Channels that transport food: digestive system (annavaha Srotas)
3. Channels that transport water and control water metabolism: digestive system (ambuvaha srotas).

Dhatu Srotas

4. Channels that transport plasma to blood and tissue: lymphatic and circulatory systems (rasavaha srotas)
5. Channels that transport blood and hemoglobin: circulatory system (raktavaha srotas)
6. Channels that nourish the muscle tissues: muscular system (mamsavaha srotas)
7. Channels that nourish the fat tissues: adipose system

(medavaha srotas)
8. Channels that supply the bones: skeletal system (Asthivaha srotas)
9. Channels that supply the bone marrow, nerve and brain tissue: nervous system (majjavaha srotas)
10. Channels that nourish and govern the reproductive tissue (in males this specifically includes semen): reproductive system (shukravaha srotas)

Waste Removal Srotas

11. Channels that carry urine: urinary system (mutravaha srotas)
12. Channels that carry feces, excrement: excretory system (purishavaha srotas)
13. Channels that carry sweat: sebaceous system (svedavaha srotas)

Srotas for the Female System

14. Channels that carry menstrual blood: female reproductive system (artavavaha srotas)
15. Channels that carry milk during location: female hormonal system

- **Elimination Srotas**: Passageways to move urine, feces and sweat
- **Female Srotas**: Passageways to carry menstrual blood and milk (female hormonal system)

Four major things can go wrong in the srota system:

Ama-based blockages are the most common form of disruption. They are a primary cause of arthritis and many other diseases, and can also be the cause of the other three forms of srota malfuncion. When the body's passageways are clogged by ama, the nearby tissues shrink, change shape or swell as in rheumatoid arthritis. Eventually the related tissue or organ could break down completely as in heart disease and hardening of the arteries. Getting rid of ama is critical to healing arthritis and other chronic conditions.

Too much material tries to move through the channels, like heavy traffic at rush hour. This can produce over-activity in the affected organs and cause symptoms such as too-frequent urination, rapid heartbeat or excessive sweating.

- The flow of materials can reverse direction or get deflected. If ama blocks a passageway, substances can back up, move up instead of downas in vomitingor move through a different srota.
- Changes in the size and shape of tissue cellse.g., tumors, moles or wartscan emerge in the srotas and related organs.

Certain types of diet and behavior can also disrupt the activity of the srotas:

- Overeating
- Eating before the previous meal is digested
- Unwholesome or incompatible food
- Sleeping after meals
- Too much or too little exercise
- Shock or concussion
- Suppression of natural urges[37]
- Excessive heat or cold
- Over worry

---

37 Charaka Samhita, Vi, V, 23.

Ama and the Doshas

The srotas are the conduits for all doshic movement. The nutrient fluid rasadhatu contains all three doshas and provides one of the ways for the doshas to move through the body. When ama contaminates rasadhatu, it mixes with the doshas and distorts their activity. As I explained earlier, the disturbed doshas flow into cells, tissues, organs and waste products and generate many forms of illness. Individual disease features reflect specific doshic qualities. Rheumatoid arthritis, for instance, can manifest in three different ways, dependent upon which doshic balance is the predominant troublemaker. The primary cause of an RA flare-up might be in the subdoshas: vyana or samana vata, sleshaka or kledaka kapha or pachaka pitta. As a result, patients could experience quite different symptoms-variations in the degree and location of pain or swelling, frequency or triggers of episodes, etc.

Ama, Digestion and Disease

Ama is the toxic product of inadequate metabolism. When food is not completely digested, a number of things start to happen:

- Step1: Ama forms in the digestive tract. If the digestive power does not burn it up quickly, the doshas will ferry it into the tissues and the srotas. When ama enters the dhatus and srotas, it triggers a series of situations which damages them structurally and functionally. They are consequensusceptible to infection and degenerative disease.

- Step 2: Ama disrupts the functions of the doshas, which leads to a deterioration in their natural modes of interaction. As pitta is disturbed, agni becomes weaker and even more ama is generated.

- Step 3: Less and less of the normal products of digestion are available to nourish the deeper tissues, and the srotas can no longer carry them properly from one tissue to the next. Specific nutrients are metabolized and absorbed at each of the seven sequential levels of tissue formation. When the process breaks down at one stage, all the succeeding stages are negatively affected.

- Step 4: Due to vata's imbalance, metabolic waste products (mala) are no longer properly expelled from the dhatus and sent to the intestinal tract for elimination from the body. As a result, dhatu structure and function are further disabled.

- Step 5: The dhatus are so blocked by the buildup of ama that they can no longer effectively take in and assimilate food and medicine. The srotas are also seriously obstructed, disrupting transportation and communication throughout the body. Regaining health can therefore be extremely difficult. If not removed through therapeutic means, ama will most likely continue to collect and cause damage over many years. Its first sites of accumulation will be those which are congenitally delicate, or are weak because of injury and/or previous episodes of ama invasion.

An MVM physician is trained to determine where ama has accumulated in the dhatus and srotas and what kind of damage has been incurred. We will also find the problem in the digestive process which generated ama in the first place.

Before we begin to analyze arthritis from the perspective of Maharishi Vedic Medicine, it is important to look at one more critical component of health and balance, namely ojas. Ojas can be understood as the first or finest layer of matter, the first materialized value of consciousness. It pervades creation and maintains the integrity of every level of the material world. When the mind transcends or associates with the unified field, ojas is produced by the body as the finest product of digestion. It is totally opposite in effect from ama, and supports every structure and function of life.

The pure intelligence or essence of the dhatus, rasa, etc., ending with shukra, is called the auspicious ojas and also called bala (strength, immunity) in the authentic text.

The more ojas we have, the healthier we are. When abundant, ojas generates enthusiasm, intelligence, understanding, a full heart, happiness, complete nourishment and health in the body and a luminous complexion. It gives good muscular development, stability, the capacity for physical work, a strong mind and refined senses. In sufficient supply, ojas also facilitates immunity.

By bala or ojas, mamsa becomes full, all movements become free and perfectly coordinated, voice and complexion become clear, and externally and internally the activity of the organs of action and the sense organs becomes self-referral, intelligent and evolutionary.

Ojas . . . is: unctuous, white, cool, stable, moving/flowing, pure in quality, soft, cohesive, and is located at the very sprouting of life (prana).

Being omnipresent in living beings, ojas nourishes every part of the body. Deficiency of ojas is equal to the destruction of the body of living beings.

Sushruta Samhita, Sutra 15: 19-22(bala).

It helps prevent diseases of both internal and external origin by maintaining balance within and among the doshas, dhatus and agni. It creates resistance to any factors which might harm dhatu structure and function.

Ojas and Arthritis

Insufficient ojas can exacerbate certain arthritic symptoms. For one thing, it can agitate vata, and agitated vata is one of the main factors in joint disorders. It can also diminsh kapha, which can also affect joint health. Decreased kapha disturbs the lubrication and binding of all the body's joints. This, in turn, produces increased looseness and dryness in the joints; weakness, pain and tiredness, or stiffness and heaviness in different parts of the body; and swelling and inflammation. Many of these widespread symptoms are commonly experienced by FMS patients. Diminished ojas can also cause obstructed or incoherent thought, speech and action; a dull, uneven complexion; laziness and lack of motivation; increased sleep; and the spread or dislocation of the doshas, which in turn can cause many types of disease.

Creating and Maintaining Ojas

The amount of ojas present in our bodies varies in relation to such factors as our doshic constitution, seasonal conditions and age. Human beings have two forms of ojas. One type exists as eight drops in the heart, and their damage or loss can be fatal. The second type is the most beneficial endproduct of healthy digestion and is diffused throughout the dhatus. Ojas is created as each dhatu is built and at the last stage of dhatu metabolism, which is shukra formation. (Shukra is the last tissue to be produced.) Ojas is associated with digestion, and diet can therefore enhance or decrease its availability. Milk, butter and ghee[38] (clarified butter) will readily generate ojas. Old or leftover food, chemical additives, food that is difficult to digest, or too much or too little food will diminish ojas.

Alcohol, tobacco and prescribed and non-prescribed drugs are among other factors that destroy ojas. Physical injury; excessive anger, grief, anxiety and thinking; excessive physical exertion or exercise; staying awake at night; and over-elimination of kapha, blood, semen or waste products all inhibit the process of dhatu transformation and consequently decrease ojas. The importance of ojas for health and even enlightenment cannot be emphasized enough. To quote Maharishi:

With the full enlivenment of ojas in the physiology, the intellect blossoms in its full (self-referral) awakening, and this is how pragya aparadha is overcome, and this is how the basis of sickness and suffering is eliminated. This is how the boundaries

---

38 The recipe for preparing ghee is given in Chapter 7.

of individualities break and this is the awakening of cosmic reality. This is why the entire purpose of Ayur-Veda or knowledge of physiology is to maintain all physiologic structure and functioning in such a way that ojas is constantly generated and maintained on its highest and supreme efficiency level of effectiveness.[39]

I wanted to give you this basic picture of Ayurvedic physiology before I described the various forms of arthritis and their treatment in terms of Maharishi Vedic Medicine. Patient education is extremely important in MVM. Both my colleagues and I have found that our patients follow both the spirit and details of the treatment regimen more readily and accurately if they know the general "whys and wherefores." This is quite important, as your health depends heavily on your participation in the MVM treatment program. Moreover, once health is regained, the recommendations we make for home treatment are vital for maintaining health. The basic knowledge I have tried to provide so far should help you understand the treatment components and make healthier choices in your daily routine and diet over a lifetime.

---

[39] Maharishi Ayur-Veda Physician Training Course I, Maharishi Ayur-Ved Medical Association, 1993, p. 40.

Chapter Seven

An Ayurvedic Portrait of Arthritis

All the different kinds of diseases cannot be apart from (devoid of) the doshas. Even so, those caused by (arising from) the abnormalities of the dhatus (tissues) cannot be without the involvement of the doshas.[40]

Remember that MVM physicians treat the patient, not the disease. We know that the various forms of arthritis and other illnesses are ultimately connected to imbalances in the doshas and the condition of agni. When we determine which doshic disturbances are the primary factors in a patient's illness, we address those imbalances first, while also taking into account the patient's prakriti, or natural doshic constitution. Consequently, although several of my patients may be diagnosed with the same disease-OA, for example-their treatment regimen may vary. The confusing array of secondary symptoms which patients sometimes experience often clear up without individual attention, as they are usually a byproduct of the fundamental imbalance in doshic activity.

Ayurveda and the Path of Disease

By the time clear symptoms emerge, all three doshas have become highly abnormal, and many secondary symptoms and conditions may develop. As a result, diagnosis and treatment can become complicated. Without Ayurveda's ability to identify the root cause of disease, a physician is stuck with trying to minimize a myriad of

---

[40] Astanga Hrdayam, Volume 1, Translated by Prof. K.R. Sri Kantha Murthy, Krishnadas Academy,

seemingly disconnected symptoms. For example, fibromyalgia symptoms are so varied and widespread that physicians are only now recognizing it as a single disease. Though it is certainly necessary to relieve painful symptoms, if the major imbalance remains unresolved, it may broadcast the seeds of future illness. Though dormant for awhile, almost inevitably the doshic imbalance will manifest again when conditions permit. This is one reason why the symptoms associated with OA, RA and FMS flare up, disappear and then reappear.

Marilyn's Story

Marilyn, a forty-seven-year-old high school teacher, as well as mother and wife, had been diagnosed with osteoarthritis, which was mainly affecting her upper and mid-back, neck and hands. Her symptoms, which had begun five years before I first saw her, were getting more severe. Digestive problems had shown up at about the same time that her arthritis symptoms appeared, and constipation had been an increasing problem for the previous two years. About a year before she came to see me, Marilyn had been told that she had a parasitic infection. She had done a lot of cleansing, but this had not changed her symptoms.

During her first visit, I observed that Marilyn's skin was extremely dry and cracked, especially on her hands and feet. She reported that she experienced crackling sounds and pressures in her ears. To an MVM physician, these were clear signs of disturbed vata dosha.

One week after her first visit, Marilyn learned the TM technique. I also prescribed an oil massage, called abhyanga, which she could giver herself at home, and a diet to strengthen agni, eliminate ama and rebalance her doshas. After four weeks, she returned to my office and stated, with relief, "I can't believe that my neck pain and stiffness have gone. I suffered for four years. My joints are still sore but the soreness is less severe. I feel more balanced. There is less anxiety and my head and my thinking are clearer." Marilyn also reported that her food and sugar cravings had almost completely disappeared and she had lost ten pounds. Her constipation had improved, but her ears still felt blocked.

After six more weeks on an MVM treatment regimen, Marilyn returned to my office and told me that she now had little or no joint pain, depending on her activity. Her skin was better and the drying and cracking had diminished. Her ears had also started to improve. Marilyn confided that she was both happy and impressed that she could feel better so quickly without experiencing any side effects. I made additional dietary recommendations, and prescribed some herbs and a deep cleansing program called Maharishi Rejuvenation Therapy. Marilyn continues to see me about every three months for a seasonal check up to prevent any potential flare-ups and maintain her good health.

Hindsight

What if I had known Marilyn for many years? Knowing about the six stages of disease, I might have been able to prevent the onset of OA altogether. To show how this could have been done, let's trace a hypothetical picture of the prognosis of Marilyn's illness through all six stages.

Stage 1. Accumulation

Marilyn lives in upstate New York, a geographical region which has long, cold, snowy winters. Suppose she likes cold drinks and ice cream and continues to consume them even when the whether turns. Aside from that, she is health-conscious. Having been told that raw fruit and vegetables are one of the best things she can eat, they are a large part of her daily diet.

Let's say that Marilyn was born with fairly strong agni and digestive strength and most of her life she has been able to eat what she wanted without obvious consequences. However, she noticed that as she got into her late thirties (a time when vata may start to increase), her digestion and elimination were not as dependable as they used to be. Sometimes raw vegetables produced gas; ice cream made her feel sluggish and cold drinks sometimes even produced a little anxiety, especially the fizzy ones.

These symptoms were not painful and only occasional, so it never even occurred to Marilyn that something might actually be going wrong. However, if Marilyn had seen me at this point and made a few changes in her diet and lifestyle, any further deterioration could probably easily have been prevented.

Stage 2. Aggravation

Marilyn's discomfort grows a little more frequent. She finds that raw food, instead of helping, produces gas. When she eats ice cream, she feels cold, even in summer. However, nothing that she is experiencing really interferes with her daily functioning. She experiments with supplements and digestive enzymes recommended by friends and figures that will take care of the symptoms. She is not yet even considering a trip to her doctor.

Stage 3. Dissemination

Marilyn's hands and feet are often cold and she wonders if she is developing a circulation problem. Her skin is dry and she starts using creams, especially on her hands and feet. She experiences bouts of restlessness and insomnia. After she eats, she often feels bloated and gas is getting more common. When she wakes up in the morning, she feels a little stiff, but a hot shower usually fixes this. Marilyn is wondering if all this is just an inevitable consequence of aging and nothing that a doctor can really help.

Even though symptoms are beginning to spread, if Marilyn came to see me at this point, I would be able to detect the growing imbalance and prescribe Ayurvedic remedies which could reverse the situation fairly quickly and simply. Vata increase is a natural part of aging. However, if an individual has a vata-dominant constitution and a vata-aggravating diet or lifestyle, vata-related conditions such as OA are more likely to develop. Fortunately, MVM has many procedures to counteract the increase of vata due to age, lifestyle and diet.

Early detection of imbalances is one of Ayurveda's great gifts. Full-blown disease is not inevitable. Caught early enough, many serious conditions, including joint diseases, can be prevented. I recommend seasonal checkups to all my patients, even when they are feeling largely healthy, as Marilyn still is at this point. MVM diagnosis can catch the subtle imbalances and reverse them before real disease arises.

4. Localization

After a lifetime of extremely dependable elimination, Marilyn is experiencing bouts of constipation. Her hands and feet are so dry that they have begun cracking, irrespective of the regular use of creams. Bloating is a regular feature of digestion, and her joints ache, especially those in her spine and hands. Marilyn has also lost her ability to concentrate and is feeling increasingly restless and anxious. Her short-term memory is also poor. She is also starting to suffer from allergies.

Marilyn still thinks this may be a product of middle age or pre-menopause. She is experimenting with various supplements from the local health food store. However, she is having so many different problems and each one needs a different kind of herb or supplement. She is told that her discomfort might be due to parasites. Parasites are certainly known to produce both digestive havoc and widespread symptoms. She tries a cleansing program that involves lots of fresh, raw food and various herbs. Since too much raw food aggravates vata, her digestion and constipation only get worse.

Finally, Marilyn decides to check in with her doctor. However, her symptoms are so general that he cannot isolate a cause or define an actual disease. His only choice is to try and control her discomfort.

He prescribes medications for her allergies and a mild pain reliever, to be used only as needed, for her stiff, achy back. He also recommends some over-the-counter medicines to help with gas.

None of these, of course addresses the doshic imbalances and toxic buildup that are now found in many of the body's tissues and srotas, distorting a large number of physiological functions. At this point, MVM can still reverse the disease process and restore health, but the time and effort involved will be greater. Marilyn will have to make adjustments in her diet and daily routine to reduce ama and balance vata dosha. She may need a few herbs and a cleansing program, or some yoga postures to help maintain joint health. However, Marilyn still does not have OA, and she can avoid it. But she doesn't. She takes the recommended pills and continues on with her life as it has always been.

5. Manifestation

Marilyn's joints are now painful. The morning shower helps, but she also finds herself reaching for the pain medication more and more often. Constipation is a large and regular problem. She feels anxious much too often and she has started feeling pressure and hearing crackling noises in her ears. She goes back to the doctor to find out that she now has an identifiable condition: OA. The doctor prescribes NSAIDS to reduce the pain and swelling in

Marilyn's joints, as well as some gentle forms of exercise and physical therapy, especially swimming.

Marilyn enjoys exercising regularly anyway, but is not excited about the possibility of spending a whole lifetime on pain medicine. Her doctor does not see the interconnection among the rest of her symptoms-ear pressure, cracked skin, etc. and only has piecemeal recommendations to ease her discomfort. Since Marilyn complains of growing anxiety and sleep problems, her physician senses that stress is playing a role in her complicated condition. He recommends that she look into stress reduction techniques and ways to reduce the pressures in her life. In a way, Marilyn feels like she is still standing in her local health food store, trying to choose among hundreds of supplements and herbs to reduce an ever-increasing number of symptoms-one or two at a time. Only the symptoms are getting worse and the prescriptions from her physician are definitely less user-friendly than most of those herbs. Some of them have some pretty mean side effects.

"How did I get here?" Marilyn wonders. "How did I get to a place in my life where I have to choose between increasing levels of pain and potentially scary, medicine-related side effects? How did I get to a place where really basic things like digestion and elimination are so "iffy" and require so much attention?"

If Marilyn discovers MVM at this stage, we can still correct the doshic abnormalities at the root of her disease. We can prevent any additional spread of the ama and aggravated doshas and inhibit the development of chronic disease or secondary diseases. Many symptoms will diminish even within a few months or weeks of starting to use MVM, but long lasting healing will probably take longer to achieve. Marilyn may also have to be on a health maintenance program for a sustained period to stabilize the doshas and strengthen her digestion.

6. Disruption

Marilyn is still trying to palliate symptoms and has not found the answer to the mystery of her many-sided problem. She can't take much in her life for granted anymore. Her spine registers pain even in simple movements. It is difficult to use her hands to accomplish even simple things like cleaning, or opening jars or typing. The most recent x-rays show the beginning of degeneration in her cervical vertebrae.

She continues trying different diets-so many to choose from-but her digestion keeps producing gas out of everything. She is hungry all the time because, due to poor assimilation, her body isn't getting what it needs. She experiences strong food cravings and puts on twelve pounds. Despite medication, her allergies get worse. She feels chronically depressed and tired, and her memory is so bad that it is interfering with her work. Marilyn is taking hormone replacement therapy, but this has not improved her memory or other problems.

If Marilyn uses Maharishi Vedic Medicine to address the broad scope of dysfunction in her mind and body, she can still find relief. Her symptoms can be comprehensively diminished and the deepest imbalances at the root of those symptoms can be normalized. Further bone and tissue damage can be prevented and the spread of secondary conditions can be stopped. It will take time and commitment both from Marilyn and her physician. She will have to make definite lifestyle and dietary changes, and invest in the appropriate herbs and cleansing programs. However, through MVM, she can stop the spread of secondary symptoms and reestablish the inner balance which is the basis for health.

Though I was pleased with her progress, I also know how much of Marilyn's pain could have been avoided if I had been able to catch and treat her imbalance earlier; or, if Marilyn herself through patient education and increased sensitivity, had been able to detect the seeds of illness in her early symptoms and had taken steps to stop them from sprouting.

Taking It all Down to the Doshas

We now have enough basic information to understand the Ayurvedic picture of Marilyn's disease, osteoarthritis. In MVM, osteoarthritis is called sandhi vata, because vitiated vata dosha is the primary culprit. The subdosha, vyana vata, is particularly involved. Vyana vata is found all over the body and governs all the body's bending and moving, from the blink of an eye to the rotation of a joint. Kapha, especially sleshaka kapha, which governs joint lubrication and cohesion and binding throughout the body, is also strongly involved.

OA comes about when excess vata builds up in the joints over a long period of time. The increase in vata can have many causes: irregular or stressful daily routine; worry, fear and anxiety; too much dry or cold food; seasonal influences; continuous exposure to cold and wind; trauma or injury. Age, however, is the most common factor. As you may remember, from about middle age onwards, vata becomes the body's predominant dosha. Individuals who have more vata in their doshic constitution or prakriti will be more vulnerable to the adverse effects of increased vata. The weight-bearing joints are the most susceptible-especially the hip and knee-as well as any joint that has been injured. Being overweight also adds to joint vulnerability.

As vata grows so does its property of dryness in the body. Simultaneously, kapha decreases and the body loses some of kapha's unctuous, lubricating qualities. Two of kapha's natural sitesthe chest and jointsare particularly affected by diminished kapha. The joints lose lubrication and dryness grows. They become weaker and start to stiffen.. As the process continues, the ligaments, tendons and synovial membranes lose strength and flexibility. Joint movement becomes painful and restricted. As kapha's unctuous attribute becomes less available, friction between the bones increases and eventually cartilage, the spongy cushion between the bones, degenerates. With the loss of cartilage, the bones rub against each other and acquire a rough surface, sometimes creating bony outgrowths called spurs. The increased dryness and friction also results in inflammation and painful, limited motion. In the long term, deformity can also occur.

With OA, because pain is largely associated with movement, it decreases when resting. However, vata increases in cold, dry and windy weather and pain may increase under these conditions. Secondary complications can include muscle strain, as muscles try to compensate for the joint weakness and pain or protect the diseased joint. Spinal spurs might compress spinal nerves, which causes extreme pain and impairs the physiological systems affected by the constricted spinal nerves. Insomnia is another possible side effect. Any vata disturbance can cause enough anxiety and restlessness to prevent sleep.

We know from MVM that OA is most often due to the increased vata which comes with age. We also know that OA can often be prevented, or at least minimized. Clearly, not everyone suffers from the painful symptoms of OA-and among those who do contract it, some get it far later in life than others.

Now that you understand how some of vata's qualities can cause damage when it is excessive or imbalanced, you can understand many of Marilyn's symptoms. The appearance of an identifiable disease, OA, was the late stage in a long term process of doshic disturbance, which affected many areas of Marilyn's life. With this knowledge, I was able to address these varied symptoms with great success, so that Marilyn recovered not only from osteoarthritis, but also from many of the other problems that she brought to my office. When people as young as Marilyn develop OA, it is likely that their prakriti is vata-dominant or that they have an inherited susceptibility. I was therefore happy that Marilyn chose to continue the maintenance program I prescribed to prevent future difficulties.

Ankylosing Spondylitis

An increase in ama and vata dosha is a key cause of spondylitis a well as OA. However, in spondylitis, ama largely impacts one particular tissue: bone, or asthi dhatu. While OA is a degenerative disease in which vata aggravation results in joint deterioration, AS involves an abnormal growth pattern in the bone tissue. One of the primary factors in OA is the natural, age-related increase in vata, but AS is related to improper bone tissue metabolism. As ama accumulates in the bone tissue, the digestive fire associated with bone, asthi agni, also becomes weaker. This further disables bone tissue metabolism and asthi dhatu manifests its increasing dysfunction as abnormal bone growth in the spine. Roughness is the vata quality most strongly expressed in this disease.

We already know that ama results from weak or incomplete digestion. Why, however, does the ama effect asthi dhatu in this case? Some weakness must already be present in that tissue which makes it vulnerable to ama, and a number of factors could be involved: heredity, previous injury, job-related strain, improper exercise which pounds or puts too much pressure on the joints and bones, emotions stored in the spine. Factors which deplete agni and debilitate digestion and tissue metabolism include eating incompatible foods; eating food which is too dry or too heavy; and eating meat frequently when digestion is sluggish.

Ama, Vata and Fibromyalgia

Fibromyalgia Syndrome involves chronic diffuse pain, as well as a host of secondary conditions, including fatigue, depression, sensitivity to physical activity, joint pain and loss of memory and concentration. Ayurveda attributes the broad range of symptoms to both widespread ama and vata. In this disorder, ama has settled in a large number of srotas and several dhatus. It is more likely to accumulate in tissues and passageways that are already weak, due to trauma and injury, misuse (too much or too little use), inheritance, previous illness, etc. In FMS, ama has circulated to such a degree that the flow of intelligence throughout the body is impaired.

Wherever ama has collected in tendons, muscles and ligaments, achiness, we feel achy, stiff and heavy. Wherever ama has blocked or slowed activity in the srotas, we feel pressure. Since the srotas run through the entire nervous system, this pressure can be felt in many places.

When the nutrient fluid carries excess vata to the dhatus, it combines with sticky ama and a murky amalgam builds up. As the mix of ama and vata collects in the dhatus, especially muscle or fat, we experience dullness, heaviness, low energy and fatigue, and varying degrees of pain. Vata is responsible for most strong pain in all disorders. When excess vata mixed with ama is found in the nerve cells, bones or bone marrow, the FMS patient is faced with deep, sharp pain in the joints and bones, loss of muscle strength and insomnia. This kind of deep pain usually stays for some time once it arises. Fluctuations in the occurrence and degree of pain in FMS are due to the varying levels of aggravated vata. In an FMS patient, if vata multiplies or is vitiated by factors such as weather changes (e.g., increased cold or windy conditions), increased mental stress and worry, improper diet (too much light, dry or cold food) an irregular routine (late nights, high pressure, too much travel) or overexertion, pain intensifies. When vata decreases, the pain also subsides.

In FMS, the pain is so widespread and so many complications are involved, that it can be extremely tricky to diagnose. For example, Stan, a fifty-five-year-old male patient, had suffered with chronic allergies, sinus problems and poor digestion for ten years. He had been put on medication for high blood pressure as well, but could not tolerate the prescription. He felt so dizzy and weak that he could no longer work. When his physicians changed his blood pressure medicine, the side effects were even more debilitating. When he experienced a bout of joint and muscle pain, he was told that he had the beginning of arthritis and FMS. He knew that conventional medicine would eventually recommend pain killers and he also knew that he could not tolerate them.

Even though his disease had progressed to the fifth stage, where Western medicine could isolate and name it, I knew that the treatment had to focus on reducing ama, strengthening digestion and balancing vata dosha. With this approach, all the symptoms that preceded the onset od FMS and arthritis would also clear up.

He responded very well and very quickly to MVM. His blood pressure normalized and his FMS and arthritis symptoms decreased. He took a one week deep balancing and cleansing program (panchakarma), which I'll describe later, and felt that all the pain had left his body. He was happy and relieved to find a medical paradigm which could affect so many complex symptoms simultaneously-no matter what name we gave them.

Amavata: Rheumatoid Arthritis

The Ayurvedic name for RA is amavata, which tells us right away which dosha is once again responsible, along with its partner, ama. The major cause of RA is indigestion or incomplete digestion, due to weak agni. Digestive capacity can be sluggish due to inheritance, a sedentary lifestyle or bad food choices and eating habits, such as:

- Eating too much heavy, unctuous food or consuming too many cold foods and liquids
- Doing too much heavy exercise after a big meal
- Exposure to cold after eating
- Eating before the previous meal has been digested
- Eating incompatible foods[41] or foods with opposite qualities (dry with moist, hot with cold, etc.)

Once agni is diminished, nothing is properly digested and ama is produced. It is absorbed by rasa dhatu in the gastrointestinal tract and carried, propelled by vata, to kapha's sites, including the stomach and joints, where it becomes even more putrified. The corrupted rasa dhatu, called amarasa, resembles what allopathic medicine calls rheum. From the stomach, amarasa travels to the heart, where it invades the circulatory system and is carried throughout the body. It vitiates all three doshas and obstructs the srotas of the circulatory system. This amarasa appears in different colors and its texture can best be described as extremely slimy. It further suppresses, the digestive power and metabolic processes and creates heavy feelings in the heart.

---
41 The next chapter explains the concept of food incompatibility in Ayurveda.

The amarasa can be the source of several serious diseases, but in the case of RA, it afflicts the joints, a seat of sleshsaka kapha. Joints where excess vata has already accumulated are vulnerable and amarasa will appreciate there. Most often, the symptoms first appear in the smaller joints, especially those in the fingers and toes. It may then progress to elbows and ankles and finally spread all over. When amarasa mixes with vataforming amavata vata's dryness makes the ama even more condensed, hard and sticky. The amavata literally gets stuck in the joints, resulting in stiffness, dullness, heaviness and swelling. It distorts functioning in both the joints and the surrounding srotas and dhatus (muscles, fat, etc.) As the amavata collects around the cells and in all the spaces between them because it is too thick to enter, swelling and inflammation arise and both vata and kapha grow more disturbed.

As a result of this pathogenic activity, the fibers of the synovial membranes loosen, and cartilage starts to decompose. Excess secretion of amarasa mixed with vitiated kapha creates edemic conditions in the already inflamed joint. In the next level of deterioration, vata's tendency to desiccate and stiffen causes the muscles to contract and harden, producing deformity in the joint. Other symptoms such as fever, lethargy, loss of appetite, headaches, hypertension, indigestion, general malaise and edema also arise as the ama spreads and all the doshas become more disturbed. Joint pain increases with the localization of amavata and greater levels of vata aggravation. Because kapha dosha is also a major player, cold, wet conditions increase discomfort.

Obviously, this picture of RA is quite different than the one currently painted by allopathic medicine. Instead of immune dysfunction-potentially triggered by infection or trauma-being at the start and heart of the disease, Ayurveda describes a long, cumulative process of development, which begins, simply enough, with weak digestive fire. Consequently, its manifestation can be stopped through preventive measures, especially if the potential for RA is detected in its earlier stages using the sensitive diagnostic tools of MVM.

Lupus

Ayurveda does not describe a separate disease similar to lupus. However, what allopathy classifies as lupus is, in Ayurvedic terms, an advanced stage of RA. The amavata has become so pervasive and thick that the disease has become systemic, spreading far beyond the joints and affecting connective tissue throughout the body. The immune system is seriously compromised as amavata spreads throughout the body, blocks srotas in all the tissues and disturbs or even destroys whole organs and systems.

Lupus patients are particularly subject to depression and anxiety because they are told that their condition is incurable and potentially fatal. In a condition in which the dysfunction is so widespread and advanced, I cannot promise my patients a complete cure. However, through MVM, I have found that patients experience long periods of remission and an overall improvement in their quality of life. Further degeneration is prevented and patients are able to substantially reduce their dependence on conventional medicines-steroids,

NSAIDS, etc. I find that offering even the possibility of remission and the prevention of additional damage brings a wave of badly needed hope and positivity into the lives of people faced with apparently incurable conditions. Conveying this gentle confidence to my patients helps turn their spirits around, and this in itself greatly assists the healing process.

Helping Karen Deal With Lupus

I have a female patient who was diagnosed with lupus about one-and-a-half years before she came to see me. A computer science student in her twenties, Karen was understandably depressed by her disease. She was looking at the possibility of a life of increasing pain and debilitation, rather than the usual things a young girl dreams abut- love, family, a successful career.

Prior to her diagnosis, she had experienced a flu-like syndrome that included muscle aches and pains and tremendous fatigue, which plagued her for weeks at a time. Her physician recommended over-the-counter anti-inflammatory agents but these did not help. After about ten weeks, she developed a skin rash on her face and the small joints in her hands began to swell. At this point her physician gave her more extensive tests and found that she had lupus. He immediately prescribed high doses of steroids. The steroids provided relief from pain, but she developed "moon face" and swelling throughout her body. She put on weight and continued to feel tired-as well as disturbed by her appearance. She dropped out of school for two semesters because she couldn't cope with the demands of her course work.

When Karen first visited my office, she was still taking steroids. I left her on the medication for awhile and started her on an MVM regimen. We focused on reducing her joint pain, strengthening her immunity, clearing the skin rashes and alleviating her anxiety and depression. In addition to the herbs, dietary and other recommendations, I prescribed the TM technique, which she learned and practiced regularly.

In just four weeks, Karen's joint pain was virtually eliminated and I asked her to work with her doctor to reduce the steroids gradually. Karen felt a deep sense of relief and confidence that she could handle her disease and overcome it. After six months on her MVM treatment program, she was completely off steroids. She had lost weight and gone back to college.

Karen has continued to make regular use of MVM therapies for the last year-and-a-half. Her disease has stopped spreading and is well-controlled. She uses a daily oil massage and the TM technique on a daily basis. She takes herbs to promote joint and muscle strength as well as immunity, and eats fresh food. Karen has also grown extremely self-aware. When she eats incorrectly for her condition-e.g., frozen or heavy food-she immediately experiences increased joint stiffness. Through our patient education program, she knows why the problem has arisen and how to adjust her diet to correct it. She is feeling genuinely optimistic about her future.

Vata Rakta: Gouty Arthritis

The doshas involved in this painful disorder are vata and pitta, and symptoms and treatment will vary, depending on which dosha is dominant. Once again, the factors trigger trigger imbalance include heredity and doshic constitution, injury and inappropriate diet and lifestyle. If an individual-especially one who is predisposed by inheritance-eats too much salt and too much spicy, sour, pungent, alkaline or fermented food, pitta will become disturbed, which creates heat in the blood (rakta dhatu). Yogurt, cheese and protein-rich foods like meat and fish, as well as alcohol and caffeine, all add to the imbalance. As with other forms of arthritis, poor eating habits have a role as well. Eating with indigestion or before the previous meal has been fully digested both cause trouble. Anger and stress also exacerbate the imbalance.

Vata gets distorted by too little sleep, an irregular routine, overexertion, suppression of natural urges and too much cold, dry food. A lifestyle with insufficient activity, that produces an unhealthy level of physical delicacy and softness, or a lifestyle with too much pressure and excitation, might also vitiate vata.

The abnormal doshas travel from the digestive tract and through the circulatory system via rakta dhatu and settle and collect in a weak and therefore susceptible joint. In this case, the joints in the toe and thumb are usually the first to be attacked, often due to previous injury or genetic predisposition. However, if not stopped, this condition can spread to joints throughout the body.

Both aggravated vata dosha and rakta-and therefore pitta-are always involved, but usually one or the other is a stronger influence. Vata dominance involves symptoms such as dryness, dark discoloration, tingling and a breaking kind of pain in the distressed joint, as well as general malaise. Stiffness and contraction will also occur in the affected joints. If rakta is the stronger factor, the patient experiences redness, burning sensations, tenderness, itching and oozing wounds. Excessive sweating and thirst might also be present. The problem can localize in the skin as well as the joints, and cause many of the same symptoms: redness, dryness, itchiness, oozing sores and burning.

Carpal Tunnel Syndrome

This particular disease begins with overuse or wrong use of arms, wrist joints and fingers, rather than poor digestion and ama. It is vitiated vata dosha which adversely affects the ligaments, but its disturbance is due to incorrect or excessive use of the hands, wrists, etc. Here, vata's qualities of rigidity, roughness and hardness build and the natural unctuous quality in the joints decreases. As vata builds, the ligaments and muscle tissue lose flexibility and harden until all movement is difficult and painful. (Remember that vata is associated with all pain.)

Now that you have a basic sense of how MVM looks at disease, we'll explore ways both to treat and prevent these and other arthritic conditions. As you will see, the focus is consistently on reducing ama and rebalancing the involved doshas. Poor diet and lifestyle are almost always sources of imbalance, and adjustments in these two areas are things we can do for ourselves with a little effort, determination and the appropriate knowledge and guidance. Consequently, we'll explore Ayurvedic dietetics and behavioral recommendations first. If we eat to create health and doshic balance and establish a daily routine that does the same, even serious problems can be corrected or ameliorated, or avoided completely.

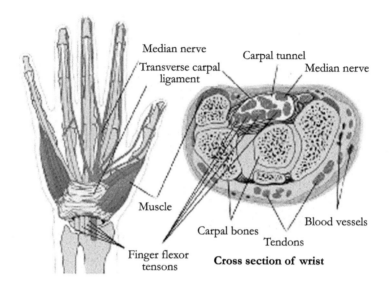

Cross section of wrist

Chapter Eight

Food and Freedom from Joint Disease

One should take food in a prescribed manner with due regard to his own self. The knowledge of the usefulness or otherwise of food articles is the sine qua non for self-preservation.[42]

In Ayurveda, healthy digestion and a good diet are critical for health. Determining the right diet eating habits encompasses many factors, including individual constitutions and imbalances. Many imbalances can be adjusted largely through dietary changes before they enter the more serious stages of disease. A consistently inappropriate diet can destroy digestive power, while the right diet does a great deal to strengthen and maintain health.

MVM's dietary recommendations are based on the ways in which each food influences the doshas. If our diet supports doshic balance, digestion will produce exactly what we need to sustain both the physical and non-physical (mind, ego, senses, etc.) aspects of life. The food we eat not only supplies the raw materials for the creation of cells and tissues but also influences the effectiveness of digestion itself.

The Two Phases of Digestion

The Ayuredic texts describe two major phases in the digestive process. The first phase, called prapaka, takes place in the

---

42 Charaka Samhita, Vimanasthana, 1:5

gastrointestinal tract and includes every activity up through absorption. When the food we consume is sufficiently broken down, it is called aharasa, as we learned in Chapter Six. It is then absorbed through the G-I tract into the circulatory system, and metabolism, the second or post-absorptive stage, called vipaka, begins. This phase, we have learned, is concerned with nourishing and building all the body's dhatus or tissues.

During prapaka digestion, which begins with eating and swallowing, food undergoes a series of conversions, called the three transient phases of digestion. Each stage is influenced by the dosha which governs the area of the body in which digestion is taking place.

Taste has a significant role in digestion, and Ayurveda describes six tastes: sweet, sour salty, pungent, bitter and astringent. Each dosha is associated with a taste and each meal should contain all six to provide complete and balanced nutrition. As food passes through each of the body's dosha-dominant zones, it takes on the taste associated with that zone, even if it had all six tastes when it was first eaten. Jatharagni initially transforms the food we eat into a largely sweet taste, as it passes through the kaphic area in the stomach. The food becomes predominantly sour in the pitta area in the small intestines, and takes on a pungent quality in the vata zone in the large intestine. At each metabolic stage, the whole body experiences the effects of the dominant dosha. For example, at the first level of digestion, kapha creates a heavy, sometimes even sleepy feeling. In the pitta-dominant period, body temperature rises and we feel warm and thirsty. In the last interval, vata generates a need for activity.

Familiarity with the details of digestion gives me clues to the strength of a patient's digestive fire and the cause and location of ama production. For one thing, if agni is strong, food will pass through all three transient stages relatively quickly, whereas weak agni slows down the digestive operations. Three factors can be responsible for this:

- Agni and/or pitta are weak.
- Ama and/or excess kapha have built up in the stomach.
- Too much food and/or too much kaphic (oily, sweet, heavy) food has been eaten

If the problem is in the pitta zone, you might experience acidity soon after eating. This indicates that the sour phase of metabolism has overwhelmed the sweet stage. The causes can include: weak agni, which allows food to ferment; excess pitta or ama; eating too much pitta (sour, hot, spicy) food. Problems in the third, or vata-dominant phase, are usually a function of breakdown in the earlier states.

The Three Forms of Taste

Taste, or rasa, has three aspects in Ayurveda:
- The natural taste of food on the tonguesweet, sour, salty, etc.which is related to the combination of bhutas or elements in that food.
- The taste acquired by food as it passes through the three, dosha dominated periods of metabolism: sweet, sour, pungent
- The post-prapaka tastes-either sweet, sour or pungent-influence tissue metabolism and are not the same as a taste on the tongue. Each dhatu is governed by a dosha, and depending on the post prapaka, dosha-related taste of a nutrient, it will either help

nourish, change or activate a dhatu. The knowledge of the long-term, taste-based influence of food helps determine both the dietary components and medicinal herbs which can rejuvenate and heal the dhatus.

The Six Tastes and Digestion

Taste tells us which elements are found in each food. Due to their elemental composition, certain tastes will increase one dosha while pacifying another. Like increases like. Food that is dominated by one element or bhuta will increase the dosha that reflects that bhuta in the body. For example, food that is strong in agni or fire will augment pitta and decrease kapha. Foods are therefore classified according to tastes which either increase or pacify particular doshas.

Taste	Elements	Doshic Effect	Post-prapaka Effect	Effect on Joint Disease
Sweet	Earth/water	Pacify vata and pitta/increase kapha	Sweet	Balances OA/ gout aggravates RA/lupus
Sour	Fire/earth	Pacify vata/ Increase kapha and pitta	Sour	Balances OA, aggravates gout /RA/lupus
Salty	Water/fire	Pacify vata/ increase kapha and pitta	Sweet	Aggravates gout/RA/lupus
Pungent	Fire/air	Pacify kapha/ increase vata and pitta	Pungent	Balances RA/ lupus aggravates OA/gout
Bitter	Air/space	Pacify kapha and pitta/increase vata	Pungent	Balances gout/ RA/lupus Aggravates OA
Astringent	Air/earth	Pacify kapha and pitta/increase vata	Pungent	Balances gout/ RA/ lupus Aggravates OA

With the knowledge of taste and its influence on the doshas, we can choose foods that restore and maintain doshic equilibrium. To nourish all three doshas, we need to eat all six tastes every day in the proportions determined by both our prakriti, or doshic constitution, and vrikriti, current imbalance. If we constantly select foods which are overloaded in one taste, we will create ama and doshic aggravation. For instance, a diet strongly dominated by sweet and salty tastes will pacify vata but aggravate kapha.

Examples of the Six Tastes

Sweet. These foods will be good for osteoarthritis, FMS, carpal tunnel syndrome (CTS) and gout, but will aggravate rheumatoid arthritis and lupus.

Most grains (wheat, rice, barley, corn, etc.) Legumes, milk and sweet milk products (ghee [clarified butter], cream, butter), sweet fruits (dates, raisins, figs, grapes, pears, mangos, coconut), certain cooked vegetables (potato, sweet potato, carrot, beet root, cauliflower, stringbean), sugar in any form (brown, white, cane, molasses)

Sour. These foods will be good for osteoarthritis, FMS and CTS and aggravate gout, rheumatoid arthritis and lupus.

Sour fruits (lemon, lime, orange, pineapple, cherry, plum, tamarind), sour milk products (yogurt, cheese, whey, sour cream), fermented foods other than cultured milk products (wine, vinegar, soy sauce, sour cabbage), carbonated beverages (soft drinks, beer, champagne)

Salt. These foods will aggravate gout, rheumatoid arthritis and lupus.

Rock or sea salt, Epsom salt, seaweed; any food to which salt has ben added (nuts, chips, crackers, other processed snacks)

Pungent. These foods will be good for rheumatoid arthritis and lupus and aggravate gout, CTS and osteoarthritis.

Hot spices (chili, black pepper, mustard seed, ginger, cumin, cloves, cardamon, garlic) mild spices (turmeric, anise, cinnamon), fresh herbs (thyme, mint, oregano), certain vegetables (radish, onion)

Bitter. These foods will be good for gout, rheumatoid arthritis and lupus and aggravate osteoarthritis and CTS.

Spinach and many leafy green vegetables (green cabbage, brussel sprouts), certain fruits (grapefruit, olives, cacao) certain spices (turmeric, fenugreek)

Astringent. These foods will be good for gout and aggravate osteoarthritis and CTS.

Turmeric, honey, walnuts, hazelnuts, legumes, certain vegetables (sprouts, lettuce, most raw vegetables, rhubarb), certain fruits (pomegranate, berries, persimmon, cashew, most unripe fruits)

Food and Arthritis: Making Intelligent Choices

Obviously, we want to do everything we can to ensure that this beautiful and intricate system for nourishing and maintaining our bodies continues to function smoothly. The Charaka Samhita, the main textbook on Ayurvedic medicine, provides detailed guidelines to help us choose the right foods and digest them well.

General Guidelines for Eating Habits and Food Preparation

- Don't eat in a rush. Food taken too hurriedly moves into the wrong passages and does not enter the stomach properly. Chew your food well. Sit quietly for a few minutes after eating.
- Do not eat too slowly. This creates dissatisfaction and you end up taking more food than you need. The food might also get cold, a cause of irregular digestion.
- When eating, eat. Stay focused on eating and avoid distractions like TV, music or lively or engrossing conversations-including phone conversations. The company and environment should be pleasant.
- Learn the foods that are best for your constitution and eat them with a sense of ease and confidence. When your physiology is balanced, you will spontaneously desire and choose foods that help you stay healthy. Until, then choose foods recommended by your MVM physician.
- Eat warm, well-cooked (not over- or under-cooked) food to promote digestive fire. Warm food is quickly digested, helps in the downward passage of vata and the detachment of kapha. Except for fruit, keep raw food to a minimum. Avoid ice cold foods and liquids.
- Make lunch the main meal of the day and keep dinner and breakfast lighter both in quantity and quality. Don't eat right before bed. Avoid yogurt and cheese at night.
- Eat the proper quantity of food. The proper quantity will vary from one individual to the next, depending on the strength of their digestion. Eat to about three quarters of your stomach capacity. Leave the table feeling neither hungry nor full.
- Eat only when the previous meal has been digested. Leave about three to six hours between meals.
- Do not eat food with contradictory "potencies." The potencies of

food are described in detail below.

- Eat in a calm, properly-equipped environment not in your car or when running from one appointment to the next.
- Include all six tastes every day.
- Do not drink milk with food that includes mixed tastes, e.g., vegetables. Drink milk only with cereal, toast or sweet food, or drink it away from a meal. Milk should never be mixed with sour foods, in particular, or with fish, eggs, radishes garlic and salt.
- Don't drink large amounts of liquids just before or within one to two hours after a meal. It's fine to sip water or other beverages with your food, but they should not be too cold, preferably not below room temperature.
- Eat fresh organically grown food, free of toxins and pesticides if possible. Avoid processed food even those in the health food stores-and leftovers or reheated food.
- The cook should be happy and love what he or she is doing. Cook in a clean, uplifting environment. The consciousness and feelings of the cook go right into the food that he or she prepares.

A Few More Facts about Food

In addition to rasa or taste, each kind of food contains certain qualities and potencies, based on the its elemental and doshic make-up. At any moment in time, the doshas in our bodies are either balanced (sama), abnormally increased (aggravated) or abnormally decreased. Exposure to or habitual use of food, herbs, environmental factors and behaviors that are dominant in particular doshas and qualities increases them. For example, eating lots of sweet food and long periods of minimal mental and physical activity produce dullness and lethargy. In addition, exposure to one quality decreases the opposite quality in the body. Exposure to dryness decreases oiliness; exposure to cold decreases heat.

The Qualities of Food, Based on the Doshas

- **Vata-dominant food** is dry, rough, cold or cool, light, subtle and minute, promotingmovement, clear and non-sticky, coarse and brittle.

- **Pitta-dominant food** is slightly oily, hot or warm, sharp, liquid, sour, promoting flow or movement, pungent and scorching.

- **Kapha-dominant food** is heavy, cold or cool, soft, unctuous or oily, sweet, steady and stable, sticky and viscous.

The Influence of the Qualities on the Doshas

Food Quality	Doshic Effect	Examples
Heavy	Decreases vata, pitta; increases kapha	Cheese, yogurt, nuts, wheat, bananas, carrots, honey, oats
Unctuous	Decreases vata, pitta; increases kapha	Dairy products, oils, nuts
Light	Decreases kapha; increases vata, pitta	Barley, corn, millet, mung beans, spices, apples, many Vegetables
Dry	Decreases kapha; increases vata, pitta	Barley, corn, millet, rye, buckwheat, potatoes, beans, honey, many spices and Vegetables
Warm (Temperature)	Decreases vata, kapha; increases pitta	All warm/hot foods and liquids
Cold (Temperature)	Decreases pitta; increases vata, kapha	All cold/iced food and liquids

Potency

Virya is the energy or potency of food and herbs and is either heating (containing fire) or cooling (containing water.) The dominant taste tells whether food and herbs will warm or cool us, and creates a fundamental energizing influence in the body. Virya essentially indicates the effect of food and herbs on pitta dosha.

Pungent, sour and salty are heating and increase pitta. Pungent is the most heating taste. Bitter, astringent and sweet are cooling and decrease pitta. Bitter is the most cooling taste.

Summary of Effects: Dosha, Rasa, Guna and Virya

		Osteoarthritis	**Gout**	**RA/ Lupus**
Dosha	Causative	Vata	Pitta/ Vata	Kapha/ Vata
Dosha	Balancing	Kapha	Kapha	Pitta
Taste	Causative	Pungent, bitter, astringent	Pungent, sour, salty	Sweet, sour, salty
Taste	Balancing	Sweet, sour	Sweet, bitter, astringent	Pungent, bitter
Qualities	Causative	Dry, rough, cold, light	Dry, rough, hot, sharp	Heavy, cold, unctuous
Qualities	Balancing	Unctuous, smooth, hot	Unctuous, cold, soft,	Dry, sharp, hot

The Mental Effects of Food

We need to look at one last factor the effect of the predominant mental guna in the food we eat: sattwa, rajas or tamas.

The Influence of Sattwa, Rajas and Tamas

Sattwic Food Creates: Long life, purity, truthfulness, resistance to disease and imbalances, strength, happiness and sense of pleasure and satisfaction; bliss	Rajasic Food Creates: Misery, unhappiness, sorrow grief, disease, accumulation of ama and blocked srotas, restlessness, inability to focus or concentrate, burning sensation	Tamasic Food Creates: Dullness, lack of energy, lack of inspiration or motivation, inertia, heaviness
Sattwic Food Is: Tasty, pleasant, moist, unctuous, stable, strength-giving, nourishing to the heart; attractive to those of sattwic temperament	Rajasic Food Is: Pungent, sour, salty, too hot or sharp, rough and dry; desired by those of rajasic temperament	Tamasic Food Is: Stale, tasteless, putrid, smelling of decay, lacking nourishment, impure, toxic; leftover; attractive to those of tamasic temperament
Sattwic food Benefits everyone.	Rajasic food aggravates joint problems characterized by vitiated vata and pitta	Tamasic food Aggravates rheumatoid arthritis and lupus

As you can now see, Ayurveda provides tremendous detail about the nature of food and its effects, all of which have to be considered when I meet with a patient. That is why, in MVM, the prescription of diet and herbal remedies is highly individualized. A number of books are now out on the market which list foods and herbs according to their dosha, virya, etc. However, self-treatment using these guidelines can be like walking into a store with endless rows of supplements. Without proper diagnosis, and a complete picture of all the factors and how they interact, we could simply be applying a band aid, or even exacerbating our imbalance.

Arthritis is a complicated illness, and patients with similar symptoms may have very different constitutional imbalances. However, the chart below describes certain foods and eating habits that can either trigger arthritic symptoms in an individual who is constitutionally vulnerable to arthritis, or produce the internal conditions (accumulation, of ama, blockage in the srotas, etc.) that can ultimately result in arthritis.

Before I list some of the behavioral and dietary factors that can precipitate joint disease, I want to remind you that we make destructive choices due to pragyaparadh, the mistake of the intellect. The disconnection from or shadowed experience of pure consciousness, Nature's governing intelligence, is behind all violation of Natural Law. When we are out of touch with the totality of Natural Law, we make mistakes which damage ourselves or the environment. Our thinking grows confused. We lose the power of discernment and indulge in unhealthy behaviors. All MVM treatment programs-especially the Transcendental Meditation technique-work to reestablish that fundamental unity with Nature's infinite intelligence.

Behavioral and Dietary Causes of Arthritis

1. Causes of Rheumatoid Arthritis (Amavat) and Lupus:
- Incompatible foods, or foods with contradictory qualities (e.g., hot and coldspicy food and ice cream or hot food with a cold beverage)
- Combining foods with opposite tastes (e.g., sweet and sour) too often
- Too much heavy, unctuous food when digestion is already weak
- Vigorous exercise after a heavy meal
- Too much cold food like cheese and yogurt
- Too much dry, cold (temperature) food or cold liquids
- Eating before the previous meal has been digested
- Exposure to cold after eating

2. Causes of Osteoarthritis (Sandhivat) and Spondylitis:
- Too much dry, cold, rough (vata-vitiating) food
- Irregular routine over a long period, including insufficient sleep
- Worry, fear, pressure, overexertion
- Too much traveling
- Over-exercise in general, or exercise that places too much weight and pressure on the joints.
- Injury to joints
- Any activity-whether through work or exercise-that produces too much wear and tear on the joints

Though repetitive activity is the primary cause of carpal tunnel syndrome, it is characterized by aggravated vata and all of the above can complicate or exacerbate this condition.

3. Causes of Gout (Vatarakta):

- Too much salty, sour, pungent, alkaline, hot, sharp, fermented food (e.g., Soy sauce)
- Too much sesame, mustard radish, potatoes, wheat, vinegar, black gram dahl
- Eating before the previous meal has been digested, or when experiencing indigestion
- Too much dry, cold food
- Toxic substances, such as alcohol and caffeine
- Too much protein-rich food like meat, seafood, yogurt, cheese
- Incompatible foods in terms of rasa and virya
- Too little sleep
- Irregular routine and/or overexertion
- Anger and/or anxiety
- Delicate, soft constitution due to inadequate activitylazy or overly luxurious lifestyle
- Heredity
- Injury that creates weakness in the vulnerable joints (big toe, thumb)

4. Causes of Fibromyalgia

- Stress in general, or a stressful, pressured, irregular routine that includes insufficient sleep
- Insufficient exercise; sedentary lifestyle
- Too much sour, salty, spicy food
- All eating habits that produce ama: eating before the previous meal has been digested; eating on the run; eating too much or too little, too fast or too slow; eating foods with contradictory qualities; too much heavy food; exercise directly after a heavy meal, etc. (See earlier recommendations for healthy eating habits.)

Though I will continue to emphasize the importance of precise diagnosis[43] for each individual, the approach to healing each form of arthritis will inevitably include balancing the doshas, ama reduction and the strengthening of agni. After patients have reestablished health, a maintenance diet which supports doshic balance, prevents ama build up and the weakening of agni in the future will most likely be recommended. I have already described which doshic imbalances play key roles in the primary forms of arthritis. The charts below are meant to give you a general idea of how to eat to rebalance these doshas and reduce ama. Remember that the food selections are based on all the factors we have just described.

Diet to Pacify Vata (When Agni is Weak)

Eat the proper amount (about 3/4 of capacity) of fresh, well-cooked, food, which is tasty and satisfying. Eat in a settled environment and at regular times, with the main meal at mid-day.

Grains
- Rice: Wholesome rice (e.g., basmati) with both the husk and inner shell removed; steamed or boiled; puffed rice; dry-fried, then boiled and made into soup; dry-fried, then steamed or boiled; light dishes made from rice flour
- Wheat (Use finely ground whole wheat flour.): Crackers, unleavened bread (e.g., tortilla, chapati); couscous; semolina; biscuits low in fat and sugar; lightly toasted bread
- Oats: Well-cooked to porridge consistency

Vegetables (well-cooked and in soups)
- Tender eggplant, white pumpkin, zucchini, cucumber, asparagus,

---

43 Chapter Twelve contains more information on MVM diagnostic techniques.

artichioke, skinned tomato, celery, small amounts of carrots and spinach, green papaya

Dairy Products

- Low-fat milk, buttermilk, goat's milk, lassi, ghee [44]

Sweeteners

- All, in small amounts, except honey

Oils

- All, in very small amounts, except coconut oil

Fruits

- Grapes (ripe and in season), soaked raisins in small amounts, papaya, pomegranate, pineapple, fig, fresh apricot, orange
- Juice from vata-pacifying fruits (ripe, sweet, juicy) apricot, avocado, banana, berries, cherry, coconut, fresh fig, plum, pineapple, peach, papaya, sweet grapes, mango, sweet and juicy apple, pear, sweet orange, date, prune, kiwi, sweet melons

Beans

- Yellow mung beans (dahl) with husk removed, prepared as a liquid soup by itself or as a soup mixed with rice

Spices and Condiments

- Cumin, ginger, fenugreek, asfoetida, mustard seeds, small amounts of black pepper, cinnamon, cardamom, fennel, cloves, salt, lemon juice, tamarind

Diet to Pacify Vata

In general, eat warm, unctuous food and warm drinks, and avoid food that is light, dry or cold. Eat a sufficient quantity. Favor the

---

[44] Recipes for lassi and ghee are offered later in this chapter.

sweet, sour and salty tastes and reduce or avoid food and drinks with pungent, bitter and astringent tastes.

Grains
- Favor wheat products, whole rice, cooked oats in small quantities. Avoid or reduce barley, corn, millet, rye, buckwheat, raw oats.

Beans/Dahl
- Favor yellow mung beans with the skin removed or red lentils. Avoid all other beans.

Vegetables
- Favor white pumpkin, zucchini, okra, artichoke, asparagus, tender eggplant, carrot, beet, sweet potato with fat, tomato, cucumber, tender radish, green papaya,, spinach in small amounts. Avoid or reduce green leafy vegetables, orange pumpkin and squash, peas, potato, sprouts, mature eggplant and radish, broccoli, cauliflower, cabbage, celery.

Fruits
- Favor ripe, sweet, juicy fruits. Sweet grapes, pomegranate, mango, papaya, sweet pineapple, banana, avocado, sweet and juicy apples and pears, sweet orange, melons, plum, kiwi, peach, apricot, cherry, raisin, fig, prune, date. Dried fruit should be pre-soaked. Avoid or reduce guava, cranberry, dried persimmon, and any fruit which is sour, dry or not yet ripe.

Dairy
- Favor all dairy products, but cheese should be soft and fresh, like the Indian cheese called panir.

Sweeteners
- Favor all sugar cane products. Use honey only in small amounts.

Oils
- All oils are good.

Nuts and Seeds
- All nuts except peanuts are good. Seeds are OK in small quantities.

Spices
- Favor cumin, ginger, mustard seed, fenugreek, asafoetida, cinnamon, cardamon, clove, fennel, small amounts of black pepper, salt, lemon juice, tamarind. All other spices are also OK in small quantities.

Diet to Pacify Pitta

In general, eat food which is not too hot and drink cool to lukewarm beverages. Favor the sweet, bitter and astringent tastes and avoid food which is salty, sour or pungent.

Grains
- Favor wheat, rice, barley and oats, and avoid or reduce millet, corn, buckwheat and rye.

Beans
- Favor yellow mung beans, small kidney beans and soy products and avoid or reduce aduki beans.

Vegetables
- Favor asparagus, artichoke, white pumpkin, okra, zucchini, spinach, chicory, cauliflower, broccoli, cabbage, green beans, celery, potato in very small amounts, sweet potato, peas, green sweet pepper, green papaya, sprouts, lettuce and tender eggplant. Avoid or reduce tomato, beet, carrot, radish, hot peppers, raw onions.

Dairy
- Favor milk, ghee, butter, sweet buttermilk, sweet lassi, cream, cream cheese. Avoid sour milk products, yogurt, cheese (especially aged and salty), salty butter, sour cream and quark.

Sweeteners
- Favor white or semi-refined sugar. Small amounts of honey are okay when not experiencing heat. Avoid or reduce molasses and brown sugar.

Oils
- Favor coconut, olive and sunflower seed oil. Avoid or reduce almond, corn, safflower and sesame oil.

Spices
- Favor coriander, cumin, ginger in small amounts, turmeric, saffron, fennel, cinnamon, cardamon and lemon juice. Avoid or reduce chili pepper, cayenne, black pepper, mustard seed, clove, celery seed and fenugreek in small amounts.

Fruit
- Favor grapes, pomegranate, cashew, banana, avocado, mango, coconut, melons, apple pear, raisin, date, fig, apricot, sweet orange, sweet pineapple, persimmon, mango, kiwi. Avoid or reduce papaya, grapefruit, sour orange, peach, sour grapes, sour pineapple, berries, cranberry, prune.

Diet to Pacify Kapha

In general, choose warm food and beverages and avoid heavy, oily and cold food. Choose a light diet, and avoid large quantities of food, especially at night. Favor food that is pungent, bitter and astringent, and avoid food that is sweet, sour or salty.

Grains
- Choose grains that are at least one year old, especially barley, millet, corn, buckwheat, rye, oats, wheat and rice.
- Avoid new grains, wheat and rice in particular.

Beans
- Everything except soy beans. Tofu is OK.

Vegetables
- Favor green, leafy vegetables, asparagus, potato in very small amounts; artichoke, carrot, cabbage, beet, cauliflower, broccoli, celery, peas, pepper, sprouts, white pumpkin, zucchini, okra (if dry-fried), green papaya, tomato, tender eggplant or radish. Reduce or avoid sweet potatoes, cassava tapioca, tubers.

Dairy
- Favor lassi and buttermilk, low-fat milk, small amounts of ghee and whole milk.

Avoid or reduce yoghurt, cream, butter.

Sweeteners
- Favor honey.
- Avoid or reduce all sugar cane products.

Nuts and Seeds
- Favor sunflower and pumpkin seeds and avoid all nuts.

Spices
- Favor all spices, especially sharp pungent ones, such as pepper, ginger, etc.
- Small amounts of lemon juice are OK.
- Avoid salt.

Fruits
- Favor pomegranate, cashew, grapes, persimmon, cranberry, raisin, fig, date, peach, apple, papaya, guava.
- Avoid or reduce avocado, banana, pineapple, orange, melons, plum, prune, mango, coconut, apricot.

Meat And Fish

You have probably noticed the absence of meat and seafood in these diets. Ayurveda does not ban the heavy proteins-Ayurveda classifies them according to dosha just like all other foods-but the diets I have just given are therapeutic and heavy proteins make the cleansing of ama more difficult. If an MVM physician prescribes a primarily vegetarian diet and you feel overwhelmed by this idea, begin by substituting poultry and seafood for red meat. Eventually, you might find you can even decrease these without strain. Try to eat heavy proteins at lunchtime, when digestive power is strongest.

We have discussed diet and digestion in depth, because of its great importance, but many other factors influence the quality of our health

Maharishi Vedic Medicine in fact uses forty approaches to help reestablish and maintain health. In the chapters which follow, we will explore therapies and self-care regimens that are especially important for either preventing or healing joint disease.

Dietary Recommendations for Specific Forms of Arthritis

Recommendations for everyone:

Sip hot water throughout the day. Avoid cold food and beverages. Never eat or drink anything right out of the refrigerator.

Avoid heavy, fatty, fried, fast and processed food as well as leftovers or reheated foods.

Eat fresh fruit and drink freshly prepared fruit juice every day.

If you are in the early stages of disease, you may notice significant changes in your symptoms within weeks. If the disease is entrenched, these dietary recommendations may have to be followed for the long term, not only to eradicate the illness but also to prevent further episodes. This may be particularly true if you have inherited a genetic propensity for these conditions.

1. Gout

Avoid all pitta-aggravating food.

Avoid hot, pungent, sharp, sour, salty food; decrease salt intake in general.

Avoid caffeine and alcohol.

Avoid all fermented food, including soy sauce.

Avoid too much protein, including meat, eggs, dahls, cheese, yogurt and seafood.)

Favor a pitta-pacifying diet (as just given), which includes green leafy vegetables, fennel, amalaberry, bitter ghee, olive oil (no sesame oil), pears.

2. Fibromyalgia

Follow the light ama- and vata-reducing diet just given.

Avoid foods and spices with sour, salty or spicy qualities.

Fenugreek and amalaberry aid digestion.

3. Osteoarthritis, Spondylitis and Carpal Tunnel Syndrome

In general, follow the vata-pacifying diet just given. Emphasize bitter, pungent food and warm,

well- cooked food. Eat asparagus and artichokes.

Include enough oil in your diet, especially ghee and olive oil.

Include amalaberry, turmeric, ginger, fenugreek, asafoetida, pepper, garlic, mustard seed, rock salt and cumin in your cooking.

4. Rheumatoid Arthritis and Lupus

In general, follow a light, kapha-pacifying diet at first. Start by favoring liquid and soupy foods, that are most easily digested, slowly progressing toward a normal diet.

When ama has been reduced-shown by decreased discomfort-and agni has been strengthened, shift to the vata-pacifying diet.

Emphasize cumin, turmeric, ginger, cloves, mustard seed, black pepper, fenugreek and garlic in your cooking.

Eat a light dinner to minimize morning stiffnesse.g., light grains like couscous, or soupy vegetables or dahl. Eat no later than 6 or 6:30 PM.

Avoid dairy products, bananas, avocados, vinegar, soy sauce.

Avoid cold food and liquids.

Golden Ghee

We've mentioned ghee several times now, especially as a food that is sattwic in nature and supports the production of ojas. Ghee is clarified butter, but its properties are quite different from those of butter: It supports all the doshas and is far healthier for you than butter. In cases where dryness (vata imbalance) is a factor in arthritis, ghee is an excellent source of oil in your diet. Where kapha is implicated, as in RA, ghee in moderation will provide oil in your diet without further deranging kapha. Use ghee as a cooking oil and anywhere you would use normally use butter on toast, etc.

Ghee is sometimes available in health food or Indian grocery stores, but you can also prepare it yourself, which is more economical. Ghee can be kept at room temperature without spoiling. To cook ghee, use unsalted butter, preferably from organic or BHT-free sources.

1. Put one or more pounds of butter in a deep, stainless steel or thick (Pyrex-type) glass pot. Cook it on medium or medium-low heat and bring it to a slow boil.. Be careful not to scorch the butter while it's melting.
2. Over the next thirty-forty minutes, the water content of the butter (about twenty percent) will boil away, and milk solids will form on the surface and on the bottom of the pan.
3. When the milk solids on the bottom of the pan turn golden brown and the liquid is largely clear, remove the ghee from the heat. Don't continue to cook the ghee beyond this point or it will burn.
4. Place cheesecloth and/or a fine stainless steel strainer over a stainless steel pan or thick glass container. Pour the ghee through

The cheese cloth slowly to strain the sediment from it. Proceed carefully since the ghee is still quite hot. When cool, pour the ghee into storage containers. Mason or other sturdy glass jars work well.

Lassi

Lassi is another item which you will find in many MVM diets, because it is an excellent digestive aid. To make lassi, mix one part fresh yogurt with one, two, three, four or five parts water, according to your taste. More water makes lassi more digestible. Add any of the following to suit your taste:

honey
sugar
ginger
cardamon and honey
ginger, cumin and salt

It is essential to use freshly-prepared yogurt, started the night before or the same morning. Otherwise, leave the lassi out of your diet. The yogurt should be not too sour and should be well-formed, or semi-solid in consistency.

Chapter Nine

Holding Health in Your Own Hands

It is in the interest of everyone, healthy or otherwise, to own this knowledge of the total range of health from individual to cosmic to maintain balance in life, the basis of good health.

... The effectiveness of Maharishi's Vedic Approach to Health lies in the ability of the programme to enliven the total intelligence of Natural Law within the physiology and thereby integrate the function of all aspects of body and mind. As a result, thought, behavior, tastes and tendencies become more integrated and balanced and spontaneously move in harmony with Natural Law, which is the basis of good health.[45]

Maharishi Mahesh Yogi

Behavior, how we live, the details of our daily routine, the input we absorb through each of our senses all these affect the doshas and health. When we are totally aligned with Natural Law, we spontaneously choose food, activity and sensory input that flows with Natural Law and supports all facets of life our individual life, our environment, the entire cosmos. Where our connection to pure consciousness is shadowed or broken, we are likely to act and make choices which damage our own lives and the near and distant environment in which we live. The treatments and lifestyle recommendations that I describe in the next chapters will all help bring your mind/body back into alignment with Natural Law so that

---

45 Maharishi Mahesh Yogi, Maharishi Forum of Natural Law and National Law for Doctors, Age of Enlightenment Publications, India, 1995, pp. 34-42

disease symptoms disappear and are unlikely to return.

Many of the recommendations I make will require that you change certain habits. They may not appear to be pathogenic habits, but if they dim your connection with pure consciousness, disturb the doshic balance and generate ama, they are indeed just that. These lifestyle changes may take some willpower at first, but as you start feeling betterwhich can happen quite quickly they will be come a permanent part of your life. Soon you will arrive at that point of inner balance where all your choices automatically support life and health.

The *Charaka Samhita* recommends that you change habits gradually. Sudden or dramatic changes produce strain.

A wise person should give up gradually unwholesome practices to which he is addicted and he should simultaneously adopt those which are wholesome. On the first day one should give up a quarter of the unwholesome practice and correspondingly adopt a quarter of wholesome practice. On the second day half of the unwholesome practice is to be given up and half of the wholesome one is to be adopted; this is to be continued for the third day also. On the fourth day, three quarters of the unwholesome practice is to be given up and three quarters of the wholesome one is to be adopted. This is to be continued on the fifth and sixth day also. The process of giving up of the unwholesome practice is completed on the seventh day. By slowly and gradually giving up the unwholesome practices and by increasing the wholesome practices correspondingly, the unwholesome practices are eradicated for good and the wholesome practices are fully adopted.[46]

---

46 Charaka Samhita, Sutrasthana 7.36-38

Daily and Seasonal Routines: Flowing With Natural Cycles

MVM recommends a rhythm of activity that keeps you in tune with the doshic changes which occur in the atmosphere on a daily and seasonal basis, and in your body, based on the digestive sequence. When your lifestyle is in tune with natural cycles, you move in harmony with the local laws of nature and the whole universe. When you are out of synch, it's like trying to swim upstream against a powerful current. The result is constant strain.

I described the patterns of doshic dominance in Chapter Five. Here is an ideal daily routine, or dinacharya, both for healing and for maintaining health.

Morning:
- Wake up early, before 6 AM if possible.
- Drink a glass of warm water, then evacuate bowels and bladder.
- Brush your teeth and scrape or clean your tongue
- Give yourself an oil massage, or abhyanga.. Details are given later in the chapter. The abhyanga is particularly helpful for those with OA or those who want to prevent it, or for any vata-related symptoms.
- Shave and clean and cut your nails.
- Gargle with sesame oil.
- Bathe or shower.
- Practice the Transcendental Meditation technique.
- Exercise according to your dosha and doctor's recommendations. (Details follow.)
- Wear clean, comfortable clothes appropriate to the season and your activity.

- Breakfast is optional. If you enjoy breakfast, eat something light like hot milk or a light cereal.
- Work or study.

Afternoon:
- Eat lunch based on your doshic constitution and digestive power, the season and climate and your MVM physician's recommendations. Lunch should be the main meal of the day. Sit quietly for five or ten minutes after you finish eating. Try to eat at about the same time each day, preferably at noon, when your digestive agni is strongest.
- Work or study.
- Practice the Transcendental Meditation technique, preferably at about the same time each day.

Evening:
- Eat dinner based on your doshic constitution and digestive power, the climate and season and your MVM physician's recommendations. Dinner should be relatively light. Avoid heavy proteins and heavy food in general, including cheese, fried food and yogurt. Eat earlier in the evening, finishing by 6:30 or 7 PM. That way your food will be completely digested before you go to sleep.
- Walk for fifteen to thirty minutes.
- Engage in pleasant activity, free of pressure or sensory overload. Avoid violent, emotional or scary movies or TV programs.
- Try to go to bed by 10 PM. If you are hungry at bedtime, try hot milk with ghee, sugar, cardamon and ginger.

Try to keep a regular routine in general: Eat, sleep, exercise, meditate, etc., at the same time each day. Be sure to get adequate sleep. Irregular routine and insufficient sleep are primary sources of vata disturbance and therefore are a definite factor in OA, RA, FMS, gout, and most every other form of arthritis.

FMS and a Healthy Routine

Though I hate to say it, one patient of mine was an excellent example of how not to live your life if you want to stay healthy. Greg was a successful entrepreneur in his early thirties, with an MBA. He worked long hours, seven days a week and ate on the run. He was virtually addicted to ice cold drinks, fast food and sandwiches made with cold cuts and other cold food. He also had very irregular sleeping habits.

A former athlete, Greg no longer took time to exercise. He spent most of his pressured life sitting in front of his computer and had gained weight. The occasional beer was his only solution to the stress in his life. To top things off, Greg was also involved in a troubled relationship. At one point, Greg's work and financial pressure increased even beyond their usually high levels. Simultaneously, he had a crisis with his girlfriend and she left him suddenly. He started experiencing tension headaches, muscle pain and stiffness and a sleep disorder. At first, he was able to relieve his discomfort with over-the-counter medicines as well as hot showers. However, after awhile, the stiffness remained all day and sitting in one position for long periods became difficult. When he finally sought medical help, Greg was diagnosed with FMS.

His physician prescribed anti-inflammatory agents, sleeping pills and an anti-depressant, which marginally helped him.. However, the side effects were intolerable and he had no energy. A friend recommended that he try MVM.

I started with some simple changes, because I knew that as a bachelor devoted to his business, it would be hard for him to learn to take care of himself. I gave him some basic dietary guidelines, including a few recipes for meals with fresh foods which he could prepare relatively easily. I took him off ice cold drinks-the most difficult adjustment for him. I prescribed special herbalized oils for massage to relieve pain and remove toxins, as well as herbs to remove the ama from his joints and balance vata. I also recommended herbs to combat depression and promote sleep and general rejuvenation.

Much to his surprise, in less than two weeks, Greg's pain and stiffness were reduced by 60 to 70 percent. His anxiety was also down. He learned the TM technique shortly after this. Within three months, his pain had almost completely disappeared and he had lost weight.

I still see Greg about every three months and his FMS continues to be in remission. He is much less tense, his pain is totally gone and he has lost more weight. He even exercises regularly, including the surya namaskar yoga exercises. The more Greg flows with Natural Law in his diet and lifestyle, the better he continues to feel.

Below are details on some of the therapies I prescribed for Greg, including surya namaskar and the self-oil massage.

Exercise

Ayurveda describes two types of exercise:
- Cardiovascular or aerobic, which enlivens muscle metabolism,

increases oxygenation, strengthens the heart and improves circulation. This form of exercise should be done regularly, if your doctor approves and if your vrikrti is taken into account. Kapha vrikriti needs lots of aerobic exercise. Pitta needs a moderate amount of heavy exercise, and vata needs relatively little. Too much demanding exercise can actually aggravate vata.

- Viyayama, which means "spending energy," takes three forms: yoga asanas, pranayama (a neuro-respiratory technique) and surya namaskar, or sun salutation—a comprehensive sequence of yoga postures. These three forms of exercise have a number of general benefits:
  - They help balance the endocrine system and refine the senses.
  - They strengthen agni and enhance rasa and rakta metabolism, which improves blood and lymph circulation.
  - They reduce stress, calm the mind and body and increase sattwa.
  - They support all the functions of vata dosha and its subdoshas.
  - They are the best form of exercise for someone with a vata-dominant constitution or vata-related disease or imbalance. Consequently, they are excellent for arthritis.

The Vedic texts provide many asanas and neuro-respiratory techniques for general health; to strengthen or heal particular organs, tissues and mind/body functions; and to relieve individual diseases. When you visit your MVM physician, he or she can prescribe the asanas and pranayama exercises that will be most useful to you, in terms of your doshic constitution and the nature of your imbalance. It is important to learn asanas from someone who understands their applications and the details of their performance, both of which can be highly specific.

Directions for surya namaskar, which is helpful for almost everyone, are given below. These postures support both prevention and healing.

The best time to practice the components of viyayama is just before you practice the TM technique in the morning and late afternoon.

Abhyanga: Oil Massage

Though this procedure may seem like a lot of work in the beginning, once you do it several times, it becomes quick and almost effortless- and the benefits are immediate and obvious. Daily oil massage is excellent for everyone, but especially during the cold, dry vata season; and for anyone with vata disorders, such as arthritis and FMS. Massaging oil into the wrists and hands is also excellent for carpal tunnel syndrome. Since everyone is potentially subject to osteoarthrits, simply due to age-related increases in vata dosha, abhyanga is a universally useful preventive technique.

1. Prepare the oil.
Unless an MVM physician has prescribed a particular herbalized oil for you, use sesame oil, preferably from organic sources. If sesame oil proves unsuitable, try olive oil or coconut oil, which is sometimes recommended for pitta constitutions. Sesame oil needs to be "cured" to maximize absorption.

Cure about one quart of sesame oil at a time. **Use low heat**, and bring the oil to about 212 °, the boiling point of water. Before heating, add one or two drops of water to the oil. The water will sputter and pop when the right temperature has been reached. Remove the oil from the heat and store it in a safe place to cool.

2. The head and neck.

Warm about 1/2 cup of cured oil to just above body temperature. Take a small amount of oil in your hands. Using an open hand rather than fingertips, vigorously massage the oil into your scalp. This is one of the most important parts of the massage. Now apply the warm oil to your face and the outer part of your ears using gentler strokes. Massage the oil into your neck, using vertical strokes.

3. The trunk and limbs.

Gently spread warm oil over your entire body, including arms and legs. Now massage the oil into your arms, front and back. Use long, back and forth strokes over the long bones and circular strokes on the joints. Massage the oil thoroughly into your fingers and palms, paying attention to all the joints. Use a gentle, circular motion over your heart and a gentle, clockwise motion over your abdomen. Massage the oil into your spine, wherever you can reach, but especially into your lower back and lumbar spine, where so many people have difficulty. Massage the oil into your legs, once again using long, back and forth strokes on the long bones and circular strokes on the joints. Be particularly thorough on any trouble spots, like knee joints.

4. The feet.

Along with the head, the feet are extremely important. Vigorously massage the oil into the soles of your feet, using the open part of your hand or the side of your fist. Massage each toe and the area between the toes.

5. Time.

The whole procedure can take from 10-20 minutes. If rushed, it's better to do a brief version (fewer strokes) than skip it all together. If you have time, leave the oil on for up to 30 minutes before bathing. Otherwise, shower as soon as you are finished.

6. Cleanup.

Wash towels separately and regularly in hot water, adding Arm and Hammer Washing Soda to your regular detergent. To prevent clogged drains, wipe excess oil off your body with a paper towel before bathing.

Speech, Action and Illness

Ayurveda actually identifies certain types of speech and action as a source of disease or imbalance. In addition, time-related errors and various forms of misuse of our senses can ultimately produce illness. The Ayurvedic texts describe three potential types of mistakes in these areas: too much, too little and destructive content.

1. Mistakes in behavior: mental and physical activity and speech.

- Excessive-e.g., talking too much; too much mental focus or pressure; improper exercise or overexertion; too much traveling; consistently irregular routine
- Too little-e.g., not speaking much or keeping silent for long periods; mental idleness or laziness; physical inertia or laziness;

insufficient exercise; Suppressing natural urges (coughing, sneezing, urinating, etc.) and functions
- Damaging content-e.g., lying, gossip, harsh and abusive speech; irrelevant speech; speech that focuses on others' faults; fear, anger, greed and other toxic emotions; sleeping on uneven places; activity which endangers life, such as physical assault, alcohol and drug use, fire, exposure to radiation or toxic environments

Certain emotions cause imbalances or exacerbate existing ones, just as wrong food does.
Vata is aggravated by fear, grief, anxiety, pressure and stress.
Pitta is aggravated by anger, irritability, overexcitement, emotional intensity and competitiveness.
Kapha is aggravated by passion, greed, attachment and jealousy.

2. Misuse of the senses.

When we take information and stimuli into our minds and bodies through our senses, it is a lot like eating. If the content of our experience (and this includes movies, music and TV) is inappropriate-excessive or over-stimulating; under-stimulating; or harsh, destructive or toxic in nature-it can trigger the formation of mental and emotional ama. This kind of ama impairs mental and emotional functioning and ultimately can cause disease.

For instance, after we hear sad or frightening news, we may keep thinking about it all day and have trouble focusing on work. Waves of anxiety may come and go throughout the day. We might also have difficulty falling asleep, or our sleep is restless and disturbed by emotional or violent dreams. Consequently, we feel physically tired in the morning and mentally grey or agitated, which in turn affects everything we do all day. If we hear bad news consistently, we might find that symptoms of OA, RA or FMS flare up or feel worse, as all these conditions are sensitive to fluctuations in vata dosha.

Examples of Misuse of the Senses

Sense	Overuse	Under-use	Toxic Content
Sight	Sudden flash of bright light Extended period of Overly-bright Light	Extended period of dim light or darkness	Seeing anything violent, or Frightening
Hearing	Loud Noise or music	Too little or total lack of sound	Cruel words, frightening news, words that convey loss, angry or violent lyrics or dialogue
Touch	Anything too Hot or too Cold	Lack of tactile experience	Assault, exposure to chemicals or pollutants, invasion by worms, bacteria or insects
Taste	Too much hot, spicy food, too much of one Taste	Lack of taste stimulation, bland food or No food	Toxic, caustic, nauseating substances
Smell	Continuous Strong odors	Lack of smells	Cigarette smoke, polluted air, chemical vapors

3. Time-related errors.

In Chapter Five, we delineated some of the natural cycles and their doshic dominance. To prevent or heal disease, stay in harmony with these rhythms—hour-to-hour, day-to-day, season- to-season. For example, if you go to sleep during kapha time, before 10 PM, your sleep will be dominated by kapha's ease and restfulness, rather than pitta's intensity. If you wake up before 6 AM during the vata-dominant hours, vata's lightness will influence the whole day's energy level. If you wake up after six, during the kaphic period, then some of kapha's lethargic quality will color the day.

Changes in climate and geography also affect you. When a dosha increases in the environment, it also increases in your body. MVM describes a number of things you can do to balance the doshas when the season's shift—changes in diet, herbs, exercise levels, dress, etc.—and this seasonal routine is called ritucharya. For instance, in the fall, when the weather cools, vata increases in your body as well as in the environment, and MVM recommends a vata-pacifying diet and regular routine for that season.

Maharishi Rejuvenation Therapy (MRT)

MVM prescribes a system of cleansing and rejuvenating therapies, called Maharishi Rejuvenation Therapy. In Ayurveda, these therapies come under the category of purification, or shodhana, which means "to go away." They help the body get rid of ama, mala and excess doshas and restore doshic balance. As a preventive tool, I recommend Maharishi Rejuvenation Therapy at the end of each season to help the body clear any doshic overload that may have accumulated due to the season (e.g., excess pitta during the summer) and any buildup of ama. The balancing influence of these therapies also helps us make the physiological transition into the next season and the changes in doshic dominance and weather patterns that accompany it.

The therapies involved have deep and powerful benefits and are also an important part of the treatment of many forms of arthritis. For instance, the first therapeutic step for amavat, or RA, is *amapachna*, the dissolution and elimination of ama. Without that, nothing else works.

Shodhana therapy reverses the disease mechanisms that move ama and aggravated doshas from the digestive tract into the dhatus. Remember that at a certain point in the disease process, ama enters and lodges in weak or defective tissues, where it undermines tissue structure and function and produces the last stages of the development of illness. The procedures used in Maharishi Rejuvenation Therapy draw ama out of the tissues, return it to the digestive tract and help expel it from the body.

Its treatments are highly specific to each patient's doshic makeup. MRT also takes advantage of the naturally occurring cycles of doshic dominance and migration, an d makes use of the activephase of each dosha to pull dosha-specific ama out of the tissues and eliminate it from the body. The doshas provide the functional connection between the digestive tract and the body's tissues the dense, solid structures that remain in the body-and mala-the natural metabolic waste products that are taken from their point of origin and eliminated. We do not expel or keep doshas; they move between dhatu and mala. They carry nutrient material from the G-I tract to the dhatus and carry unusable substances away from the dhatus and back to the G-I tract for elimination. The G-I tract is the site for both the creation and expulsion of ama. The doshas provide the dynamic bridge between the G-I tract and the bodys organs and tissues. Vata dosha governs all movement and is therefore the key player in all this activity. Normalization of vata is therefore a primary objective of MRT.

Three Stages of Treatment

Maharishi Rejuvenation Therapy has three stages:
- Purvakarma, the preliminary purification procedures
- Pradhanakarma, the core of the treatment, or the five primary procedures for purification and balance
- Paschatkarma, post-treatment procedures to assure restoration of strong digestive agni and to nourish, strengthen and balance the physiology

I. Purvakarma: Preparatory Treatments

1. *Amapachana*
Dissolving and clearing ama with diet and herbs. This phase must precede any further treatment.

2. *Snehana* (Oleation)

Internal treatment
Patients take prescribed amounts of ghee or special herbs to soften and loosen ama. Ghee reaches every cell in the body, including the brain cells, and helps dislodge impurities. Its unctuous qualities are

excellent for disorders that are caused or complicated by vata, such as OA and FMS, and for dryness and anxiety.

External treatment/massage

Abhyanga. This massage uses warm sesame oil, prepared with special herbs that address the patient's specific imbalance. The nature of the massage and the herbalized oil facilitates the oil's absorption through the pores of the skin and into the dhatus, where deeply stored toxins are then dislodged.

The massage is generally given by two technicians working in synch on both sides of the body. Touch is the one sense found all over the body and this style of massage soothes the entire physiology. Touch is registered by the brain and the orderly nature of abhyanga promotes integration and orderliness in brain function. The oil is also particularly good for normalizing vata, which is associated with the sense of touch. When vata is soothed, pitta and kapha also benefit.

Deeply lubricating, abhyanga is excellent for arthritis, as it overcomes vata's drying effects as well as eliminating vata-related ama. Remember that you can do a simplified version for yourself every day at home.

Udvartana: This massage is particularly good for kapha imbalances. The oil is treated with herbs and ground grains to form a paste. It deep-cleans the skin, promotes weight loss and increases circulation to the deeper tissues.

Pizzichilli: Two to four technicians pour warm, herbalized oil all over the patient, while gently massaging the oil into the skin. The oil thoroughly penetrates the tissues, eliminating deep imbalances throughout the musculoskeletal system. It is a powerful treatment for pacifying vata and therefore excellent for all forms of arthritis and FMS.

Shirodhara: Warm, herbalized oil is poured in a continuous, light stream back and forth across the forehead. This produces profound relief from worry and anxiety-a primary cause of vata aggravation-as well as deep relaxation and coherent brain functioning.

3. *Swedana*/Heat or Fomentation Treatments

These treatments remove impurities from the musculo-skeletal system and are particularly important for all forms of arthritis. Heat softens ama, making it easier to dislodge it from the tissues for elimination. Heat also opens the srotas so that the loosened impurities can move out of the body.

- Herbalized steam opens the srotas and impurities move out through the dilated sweat channels.
- *Pinda Swedana.* Cloth pouches containing herbs, rice and milk are massaged into the body. This treatment nourishes and balances tissues and decreases pain, inflammation and swelling in the joints and throughout the neuromuscular system.

II. Pradhanakarma. These treatments are designed largely to eliminate aggravated doshas.

1. *Nasya.*

This therapy benefits, the head, neck, sinuses and shoulders. It includes two types of inhalation therapy: herbal drops and herbalized steam. Nasya clears the nasal passages and eliminates mucous from the lungs and sinuses. It is extremely helpful for kapha imbalances, increases clarity and balance in the brain and senses, and helps thyroid function. It can also release negative emotions stored in the respiratory tract.

2. Virechana. Laxative Therapy.
The patient takes a warm bath to dilate the srotas so that the loosened impurities can move from peripheral areas of the body into the intestinal tract. A mild laxative, such as castor oil or other herbs, is then used to help expel them from the body. Virechana is particularly effective for getting rid of excess pitta, which is found in the stomach, liver and pancreas.

3. Basti: Intestinal Cleansing
Basti is the most important treatment for vata-related illness, including constipation, back pain, gout, FMS, arthritis, etc. It helps with many neuromuscular disorders as well. MRT generally uses two main types of basti:

(A) Shodhana-cleansing. All the massage and thermal treatments remove ama and excess doshas from the srotas and dhatus and move them into the intestinal tract. This elimination basti uses herbalized oils and other formulas to flush all the toxins and malas from the intestinal tract and out of the body.

(B) Anuavasan-nourishing. Herbalized oils nourish and lubricate not just the colon but all the dhatus. This deeply lubricating basti pacifies vata in its own site, the colon and pelvic area.

Several external bastis are also used as needed. One, called katti basti, which means "retained on the back," applies medicated oils in a container of black gram dough which is built around the lumbar-sacral region of the spine. This helps with muscle spasm and rigidity in the lower back and strengthens the bone tissue in that area.

4. *Vamana*. Emesis.

III. Paschatkarma: Post-Treatment
Once the cause of disease has been removed through the shodhana, or cleansing procedures, the dhatus can begin to rebuild themselves. The follow-up procedures facilitate this process and assist in the reestablishment of strong, healthy digestion. After MRT, the digestive fires must be rekindled and the doshas pacified, so it is important to respect this vulnerable time for the body and facilitate a stress-free transition back to normal activity. Your MVM physician will give diet and lifestyle recommendations that will ensure that digestive strength is fully restored and that your reentry into activity supports the healing features of your treatment. These prescriptions to help rekindle agni, especially through diet, are called *samsarjana*.

Paschatkarma also involves special herbal combinations called *rasayanas*. In addition to helping stabilize the benefits of MRT, herbs and rasayanas are used extensively in the treatment of arthritis and most other diseases, and we will be discussing this in the next chapter.

Just after MRT, your cooperation with the balancing and building process going on inside greatly influences the potential for long-lasting benefits from this treatment. However, I hope this chapter and the chapter on diet have helped you see how much of the possibility for health you hold in your own hands every day. I described the Transcendental Meditation technique to you earlier in the book. The TM technique is such a powerful tool for aligning your consciousness with Nature's infinite intelligence, that if you make it a part of your daily life, you will find that making the right choices becomes effortless and automatic.

The TM-Sidhi Program

In addition to the TM technique, Maharishi Vedic Medicine offers many other programs to support genuine health, a function of fully developed consciousness. I frequently recommend the TM-Sidhi program, which you can learn after practicing the TM technique regularly for several months. While the TM technique reconnects our individual consciousness with its source in Nature's infinite intelligence, the TM-Sidhi program enhances our ability to think and act from that level. It greatly strengthens mind-body coordination and integration.

Research on the TM-Sidhi program shows that the brain experiences high levels of coherence during the practice. When used regularly, this technology is a formidable tool for rapidly creating that perfect alignment with pure consciousness which supports balanced functioning at every level of the mind/bodylife-supporting choices in all areas of behavior; freedom from stress, negativity and toxic emotions; and a joyful, open, creative and enthusiastic approach to life.

When practiced in a group, research repeatedly shows that this technology enhances not only individual life but also the life of society. Just as the TM and TM-Sidhi programs reduce stress, produce coherence and enhance health in individual life, their collective practice does the same for the environment. More than thirty studies show that group application of the TM-Sidhi program decreases incidents of crime and violence (including war-related violence) accidents and hospital admissions. For example, in 1993, 4000 people from around the world gathered in Washington, D.C. to demonstrate the benefits of group practice. The crime rate dropped significantly during this period and the decrease could not be attributed to any other interventions. In fact, it occurred during a time of intense heat which usually causes crime increases.

The concept of health in MVM includes the environment in which we live. Breathing toxic air and drinking polluted water is without question physiologically challenging. Streets, workplaces or homes polluted by stress and toxic emotions, like anger, fear and greed, also challenges our internal balancing mechanisms. The use of the TM and TM-Sidhi practices in daily life, especially in a group, can create an environment for ourselves, our families, our society, which supports health and a quality of life which we are all seeking.

Chapter Ten

Herbs and Rasayanas: Healing Gifts From the Plant Kingdom

...[E]very state of physiology has a corresponding state of inner intelligence. This is true in the case of the human physiology and it is also true in the case of the physiology of plants. Considering the physiology of a plant, there is the physiology of the root, stem, leaf, flower, and fruit; at each level the inner intelligence has a specific quality.

... When the knowledge of Natural Law is properly applied, the matching quality of intelligence within the physiology and within the plant will create a balancing effect, and the balanced functioning of the physiology will be restored.[47]

Maharishi Mahesh Yogi

Almost invariably, herbal supplements are an important part of my recommendations to patients. The herbal combinations that I prescribe are prepared by Maharishi Vedic Medicine according to the exact formulas found in the Vedic texts. The ancient knowledge of herbs is called dravyaguna, which means "qualities of matter." Dravyaguna is an extremely precise and comprehensive science that studies the name, form, qualities and uses of plants and their preparations. It covers the medicinal application of thousands of plants; how they work alone and in combination, or synergistically; detailed instructions on how they should be prepared; and equally careful instructions on how they should be taken.

---

[47] Maharishi Mahesh Yogi, Maharishi Form of Natural Law and National Law for Doctors, Second

The plant kingdom emerges, like the rest of creation, from Nature's infinite intelligence. Sound is the first and subtlest expression of each component of creation Each individual expression of consciousness has a unique vibratory structure, and consequently every herb expresses a special vibratory pattern.

Plants have a marvelous connection with human life in that each part of the human mind/body has the same vibratory quality as a particular herb. The herb which Ayurveda would describe to heal a joint, for instance, would have the same vibratory pattern as a healthy joint. When we fall ill, it means that the vibratory nature or essential frequency pattern of some physiological component or system is disturbed. The right herb will help reestablish the natural frequency in the disturbed area, resonating with that area much like a tuning fork.

Herbs match up with the human physiology in other ways as well. The manifestation of pure consciousness into the various forms with which we are familiar takes place in the same steps everywhere and for everything. Consequently, the doshas, the elements, etc., are present in plants. For example, some plants are primarily kaphic. They have abundant growth and sap. They are heavy and succulent and contain a lot of water. Vata-dominant plants have minimal foliage. They can be gnarled and crooked, or have cracked bark. Pitta plants are full of color and have brightly-colored flowers. Their sap is moderate in quantity and may be poisonous. Kaphic conditions are often treated with the root and bark of plants (dominantly earth and water). Flowers (fire dominant) are frequently used for pitta and leaves and fruits for vata. The quality of soil and the nature of the climate in which plants are grown and their doshic and elemental composition also influence their medicinal properties.

Plants, like human beings, are composed of seven dhatus or planes. The sap, for instance, is a plant's plasma and the resin is its blood. The gum is its fat, the bark is its bone, etc. The dhatus of the plant will work on the corresponding dhatu in us. Seeds are used to treat congenital diseases because of their reflection of the "seed" from which we spring.

Herbal Compounds: Creating Wholeness

In addition to the highly specific applications of single herbs, the Vedic seers saw that certain herbs increased each other's effectiveness. The addition of the right herbs make the nutrients and intelligence of a plant easier for the body to absorb and use. Ayurvedic compounds can be elaborate and involve as many as fifty different herbs. They will usually contain a core herb which targets the disease, and additional herbs with similar properties that make the primary herb easier for the body to assimilate. The complementary herbs also help eliminate waste matter and balance the effects of the main herb so that no imbalances of any sort appear. Working together, they create a wholeness that cannot be totally appreciated just by describing the parts.

I am always amazed by the comprehensive effects of the herbs. They restore health at the deepest level of physiological operation, the level of Nature's governing intelligence, and at each related level of structure and function. They work in five basic ways:

1. **Cleansing the Srotas.** Herbs are classified according to the body's sixteen systems of srotas. Each herb or compound will clear ama and impurities from one of these systems. Since the srotas provide the pathways through which the herbs reach the cells, they must be cleared first.
2. **Balancing the Doshas.** The doshic and elemental properties of the plants are used to normalize doshas and subdoshas.
3. **Nourishing and Rebuilding the Dhatus.** Each herb is related to a dhatu and this connection provides another level of classification for Vedic compounds. When one of the body tissues needs to be restored, a dhatu-specific herb is selected.
4. **Enhancing Digestion and Increaing Ojas.** Agni, one of the five universal elements, is of course also present in plants, as the agent of photosynthesis. Through agni, plants transform sunlight into life. Plants can give us their agni-their power of digestion and transformation-to enhance our own. Strong digestion clears ama and/or prevents its creation. When digestion is healthy, ojas, its most refined product, increases. Remember that ojas has widespread positive effects on health, including greater immunity, strength, and happiness.
5. **Restoring Nature's Intelligence.** The intelligence in an herb is matched with the intelligence in the body that is diseased or disorderly. The frequency pattern that embodies the intelligence in the plant resonates with the diseased part of the body and restores or reawakens a healthy frequency pattern in that area of structure or function. Herbs in the Vedic pharmacy are additionally categorized according to the same factors as food:
    - Tastes (rasa)
    - Quality (guna)heavy, light, dry, oil, etc.

- Potency (virya) heating or energizing vs. calming and cooling
- Post-digestive effect (vipaka) sweet, sour or pungent
- Unique action or characteristic (prabhava) cleanse, eliminate, nourish the muscles, build bones, etc.

Choosing the Right Herbal Formula

Fortunately, many, herbs are available to help arthritis patients. I list a few examples for you, to give you a sense of their scope. However, I ask you to remember that Ayurvedic diagnosis and prescription is based on your unique, personal constitution. Selecting an herb or herbal compound is not like going into a health food store and selecting a vitamin here or there that you think you may need. Ayurvedic herbs are both disease- and person-specific. When they work together to create wholeness, the science of their synergy is exact. Each herbal compound balances without creating side effects. It is therefore best to have an MVM physician select the herbal formulas that will really help you.

Our prescriptions also include the right time of day to take the herbs and anything that you should take with it. An anupana is a nutrient material, food or liquid, which helps carry the herb where it needs to go. Anupanas strengthen the effect of herbs and balance their side effects. They include substances such as ghee, milk, water and honey.

Herbs for Arthritis

Methi **(Fenugreek):** Promotes digestion.
Marichi-phalam **(Cayenne):** Stimulates digestion and circulation,

dispels cold, burns toxins from the colon. It is rajasic, or mentally stimulating and best for short-term use.

Karpura **(Camphor):** Enhances medicated oils, especially sesame oil, and works as a counter- irritant for muscle pain.

Marichi **(Black Pepper):** It strengthens agni and is a strong digestive stimulant. It burns up ama and purifies the digestive tract.

Shatapushpa **(Fennel Seeds):** They strengthen agni and digestion without aggravating pitta.

Sunthi **(Ginger):** Ginger is one of the most sattwic of the spices and herbs and is considered a universal medicine. Fresh ginger helps all vata disorders, while dry ginger is better for reducing kapha.

Hapusha **(Juniper Berries):** Dispels excess vata, promotes digestion, decreases kapha. It can be used as an external paste to decrease arthritic swelling.

Nagadamani **(Mugwort):** Helps relieve aggravated vata conditions like arthritis, and nervous conditions related to obstructed vata.

Tumburu **(Prickly Ash):** This is a powerful herb for eliminating ama. It destroys ama in the G-I and is particularly good for vata imbalances and arthritis. To combat RA, it works well with juniper berries. To promote digestion, it works well with ginger.

Dwipautra **(Sarsaparilla):** It helps strengthen agni and expel excess vata from the colon. It also helps relieve rheumatic inflammation.

Tila **(Sesame Seeds):** Sesame seeds rejuvenate a vata constitution and benefit bones and teeth. Sesame oil is frequently used for abhyanga.

Haridra **(Turmeric):** A natural antibiotic, it promotes healthy digestion and improves intestinal flora.

Parijata: A bitter juice used to relieve sciatica and chronic fevers and expel intestinal worms.

Syonaka: A hot, bitter, astringent bark used to treat RA.

Dashamoula: It helps all three doshas, but especially vata.

Guduci: A bitter rasayana which pacifies pitta and is used in the treatment of gout. Bala (Indian Country Mallow): A general tonic for vata disorders. It nourishes the nerves and soothes arthritic pain.

Guggul (Indian Bedellium): One of the best medicines for chronic arthritic conditions. It pacifies both vata and kapha, and is often used with small amounts of other herbs which direct its healing properties.

Haritaki (Chebulic Myrobalan): An excellent rasayana, it removes congested vata and balances it.

It feeds the brain and nerves, regulates the colon and strengthens digestion and absorption.

Pippali **(Indian Long Pepper):** Closely related to black pepper, pippali is a strong digestive

stimulant. Quite hot, it dispels cold, congestion and ama.

Medicated Oils

Lubrication is an important antidote to the vata aggravation associated with arthritis. Consequently, herbalized oils can significantly help both in its prevention and cure. MVM uses exactingly prepared herbalized oils which remove ama from the skin and permeate the tissues, eliminating obstructions and ama from the dhatus, doshas and subdoshas. These oils are used extensively in Maharishi Rejuvenation Therapy, where both the type of oil and the herbs which are added are carefully prescribed for each individual. The oils remove weakness and also purify, eliminate blockages and decrease pain.

Many types of herbal compounds have been developed by MVM to help joints. They are available as Maharishi Ayurveda rasayanas and herbal formulas, some of which can only be prescribed by an MVM physician. Two formulas available to the general public are described below:

Joint Soothe 1, a tablet, strengthens joint function, digestion and metabolism. Some of its contents include guggula, garlic, ginger, rasna (Pluchea lanceolata), ashwaganda, shilajit (mineral pitch), elephant creeper root, bishop's weed, butterfly pea and costus root.

Joint Soothe 2, an herbalized oil, contains over seventy-nine herbs and takes many days to prepare. It combines two traditional oils:

    i. Mahanarayana oil consists of sesame oil and milk cooked with fifty-six herbs on a low fire for many hours. This method of preparation preserves the potency and intelligence of all the ingredients. Mahnarayana oil improves circulation around the joints.

    ii. Vishagarabh oil contains sesame oil processed with twenty-three herbs, including staff seed oil, oil of terebinth, camphor, Indian sweet fennel, and eucalyptus oil. When used in massage, it rapidly penetrates the pores of the skin and heats the channels of circulation where it has been applied. This facilitates the disposal of ama and toxins and lubricates the joints.

Aroma Therapy

Aroma therapy makes use of the intelligence of plants in yet another way. Maharishi Aroma Oils use a synergistic combination of herb and flower extracts and the sense of smell to reestablish health. Some of the oils balance the individual doshas, while others increase joint and muscle flexibility, strengthen digestion, relax the muscles and reduce the tendency to worry, all of which are helpful for arthritis.

The sense of smell affects the limbic area of the brain which is associated with memory and emotions. Aroma therapy is thus well-suited to help with emotional as well as physical problems.

Rasayanas

Certain herbs and herbal compounds are classified as rasayanas, or "holy healers." They may contain as many as fifty different ingredients, each of which has been harvested and prepared exactly as prescribed by the meticulous science of dravyaguna. As with all herbal compounds, they help reset the biological intelligence in a particular area of the body. They increase ojas and enhance physiological strength and immunity. They also promote longevity, youthfulness, increased intelligence and sattwa. They are used to rebuild the system after the cleansing or shodhana phase of Maharishi Rejuvenation Therapy.

The rasayana which I recommend almost universally-for prevention, as well as cure-is Maharishi Amrit Kalash (MAK), which consists of two complementary compounds: MAK-4 and MAK-5. MAK was developed collaboratively by three of India's most prominent Ayurvedic physicians and herbalists: Dr. V.M. Dwivedi; Dr. Brihaspati Triguna, former president of the All- India Ayurvda Congress; and Dr. Balraj Maharishi, who trained in the Himalayas for more than forty years and worked with over 6000 medicinal plants.

Amrit Kalash means "vessel of immortality," and is the most acclaimed rasayana in the Ayurvedic pharmacopoeia. It contains more than two dozen herbs and dried fruits, some well-known-e.g., licorice and cinnamon-and some quite rare, such as heart-leaved moonseed and Bengal quince. Research has shown it to be a powerful free-radical scavenger;[48] in fact, a thousand times more effective than vitamins C or E. It has been found to help in the prevention and treatment of cancer and the reduction of chemotherapy's toxic side-effects, to greatly enhance immunity and to ameliorate many chronic diseases, including arthritis.

Each plant on earth expresses specific qualities of Nature's infinite intelligence, just as each person does. With their awesome depth and clarity of consciousness, the Vedic seers were able to perceive and identify the qualities of intelligence and the composition of the subtle elements of creation which define each plant's healing gifts. They matched up the intelligence of thousands of plants with the aspects of physiological intelligence that orchestrate the countless activities, systems and structures-large, subtle and minute-throughout the mind/body.

Every time you consume a plant or herb, you absorb its intelligence, or that aspect of Natural Law embodied in its frequency pattern, as well as its doshic and elemental makeup. When correctly prescribed, this plant restores the memory of the correct vibrational pattern in a particular area of your mind/body where it has become distorted. That aspect of your mind/body can once again resonate in harmony with the wholeness of your physiology and the wholeness of the cosmos.

---

[48] Free radicals are chemically unstable molecules which are a normal byproduct of metabolism, but can be highly destructive if their accumulation is unchecked. They are absorbed from the environment in many common ways: air pollution, pesticides, processed food, cigarette smoke, to name a few. When produced in excess, they damage things as vital as DNA, proteins and the lipids in cell membranes. Researchers currently link them to most chronic diseases, including arthritis.

Chapter Eleven

Ever-Increasing Possibilities

When the total intelligence of Natural Law-Veda-is lively in the individual physiology, there is perfect synchrony between the functioning of the individual cell and the holistic functioning of the body as a whole, and between individual intelligence and Cosmic Intelligence. With this complete integration, all thought and action are spontaneously in harmony with Natural Law and the individual enjoys perfect health. [49]

Healing With Sound-Maharishi Vedic Vibration Technology

We know now that the finest level of creation is the subtlest value of sound. We also know from our introduction to the Veda-Veda 101- earlier in this book that everything in creation has a specific frequency pattern which is a kind of blueprint for its form. These frequency patterns are the language or sounds of the Veda and the Vedic Literature. They are the intelligence which structures our mind/body and everything in our created universe.

In the last chapter we also learned that in Ayurvedic pharmaceutical science, the vibrational pattern of a plant can resonate with the same pattern of biological intelligence in our bodies to restore health. If we take this line of thinking one step further, we will find the Maharishi Vedic Vibration Technology (MVVT)-which holds out a

---

[49] Maharishi Mahesh Yogi, Mahrishi Forum of Natural Law and National Law for Doctors, op. cit., P.11.

new avenue of hope for healing arthritis and many other chronic conditions.

I remember some years ago hearing Maharishi Mahesh Yogi say that ultimately healing would be accomplished simply by hearing the Sanskrit name of an herb, because the Sanskrit sounds in a name are the first expression of the form inherent within it; i.e., the plant would not even need to be ingested. MVVT is something quite close to this. Practitioners of MVVT use specific Vedic sounds that resonate with the vibratory pattern of intelligence in diseased or disorderly parts of the mind/body. In so doing, they reestablish the original and natural frequency pattern for that area of life, and its connection to the underlying wholeness, the field of Natural Law. The result is health and a freedom from pain which is often accomplished quickly-within minutes-even with longstanding difficulties.

One woman with twenty years of neck pain and occasional immobility, who had been seeing chiropractors regularly, reported a ninety-five percent improvement. A man whose right foot had been paralyzed in a car accident hadn't felt anything in his foot for thirty-eight years. He reported, "I started feeling tingling sensations during the first session. In various parts of my foot there is much more feeling now, and walking is smoother... My ankle had been frozen at a 90-degree angle, but now there's much more feeling in the ankle, much more life."[50]

---

50 Fairchild, Jim, "Maharishi Vedic Vibration Technology: More Than Just Relief," in Enlightenment,
Vol. 2, Issue 3, Maharishi Vedic Education Development Organization, Antrim, N H, September, 1999, p. 9.
Vol. 2, Issue 3, Maharishi Vedic Education Development Organization, Antrim, N H, September, 1999, p. 9.

An Iowa woman in her mid-fifties had been experiencing pain and numbness in her hip and thigh for many years. She had almost resigned herself to a sedentary lifestyle with minimal physical movement when she went for a treatment. At the end of the first session, she found increased flexibility. She now has normal movement and is capable of the dynamic life she had been missing. An elderly, wheel-chair-bound victim of RA in Lexington, Kentucky, tried MVVT for relief from chronic pain and the chronic anxiety that accompanied it. At the end of the first treatment, the woman reported both decreased tension and an influx of happiness-and the cessation of pain for the first time in over forty years. [51]

Instant Relief from Arthritis

In the first six months of 1999, some 2000 MVVT treatments were given to people in forty North American cities. Most of the conditions addressed were long term, averaging fourteen years. Within four to five days of treatment, sixty-three percent of the patients reported between twenty-five and 100 percent improvement in their symptoms.[52] Another study, on 176 arthritis patients, used a double-blind, controlled experiment. Findings included a highly significant reduction in pain and stiffness and improved range of motion. Analysis of sub-categories of arthritis-peripheral arthritis, painful spinal disorders and rheumatoid arthritis-also showed significant results.

---

51 Erickson,
52 Erickson, Rolf, "Silent Transformations," in Enlightenment, Ibid., Pp.11-12. R., Ibid., P.11.

Results of One Step (A Few Minutes of Treatment)

Number Treated	176	Length of Time Problem Existed		
Relief from Pain:		10-41 Yrs	3-9 Yrs.	0-2 Yrs
100 % Relief	64	23	30	11
80% Relief	42	20	14	8
60% Relief	21	11	6	4
Less than 40%	31	15	5	11

Arthritis and MVVT[53]

Both the subjective reports and the initial research in the U.S. and Europe indicate that MVVT can provide striking and prompt relief for arthritis and many other chronic conditions. It may sound impossibly simple after all the complicated and time-consuming treatments you may have tried. We're not used to things being that easy, especially if we have been in pain for some time. However, simplicity is a characteristic of that most profound and orderly level of life at which MVVT works.

Maharishi Gandharva Veda

Maharishi Gandharva Veda, the traditional music of India, provides another useful and simple, sound-based therapy. The musical patterns or ragas that compose Ghandarva Veda express the laws of nature which are lively at different times of day. They reflect the different qualities (doshas, elements) in the atmosphere as the sun moves through the sky.

---

53 Study quoted from website: www.vedic-health.org.

Each raga, or melody, in Ghandarva Veda is meant to be played at a particular time of day. It embodies the impulses of Natural Law for that period and brings both the listener and the environment into alignment with those impulses. The ragas neutralize stress both in your physiology and in the atmosphere around you. If you play them in your home or office (CDs and tapes are available) even when you are not there, they will create harmony in the environment. Maharishi Gandharva Veda is also used in clinical settings to balance the doshas.

Maharishi Yoga Asanas

Asanas are defined as "sthir-sukham asanam," or postures for stability and steady, settled awareness. They provide a mild form of exercise which is ideal for vata constitutions, but benefit everyone. They can gently help increase range of motion in stiff joints and flexibility in strained or tight muscles. Certain asanas also open the srotas and therefore facilitate the elimination of ama, which is so vital to healing arthritis.

As with all MVM technologies, asanas have precise applications and rules for use. A great variety of postures are available both to prevent and treat illness in every tissue, organ and physiological function. They can also be dosha-specific and therefore used to correct doshic imbalances. The sun salutations described in Chapter Nine have comprehensive benefits effects and are recommended for everyone, healthy or not. Many other asanas are also recommended for arthritis. Asanas involve precise postures which must be learned and performed correctly to gain their full value. Maharishi Vedic

University offers an excellent introductory course on yogasanas, in addition to any special ones that your MVM physician may recommend.

Pranayama: Neurorespiratory Therapy

Prana is best defined as the body's vital breath, or life-energy. It activates both mind and body and is responsible for our higher cerebral functions, as well as motor and sensory activities. Prana permeates the air and breathing provides a constant exchange between our internal prana and atmospheric prana. Prana is subtler and livelier than the oxygen which we normally associate with breathing. It's like a fine oil which reaches every tiny part of the machinery. Pranayama is a series of powerful breathing exercises that clears the lungs, heart and all the hollow organs. It also helps propel the doshas into the digestive tract where they can be eliminated. We have eight basic types of pranayama, each of which is designed to help particular mind/body functions. I often prescribe one or more of these exercises for my arthritis patients because they can significantly improve digestion and elimination, create calm, generate coherent brain function and regulate neurorespiratory function as a whole.

Pranayama is also extremely easy to learn and do, even for people in pain. However, the exercises are quite potent, and they must be learned properly or they can actually create disease. The best time for pranayama is just before you practice the TM technique.

Maharishi Vedic Architecture: Sthapatya Veda

The truth is that the individual is cosmic on both levels-on the level of intelligence, or consciousness, and also on the level of his body, which is the expression of his consciousness, or intelligence. Because of this cosmic status of the individual, in order for the individual to be in peace and harmony within himself, everything about him should be in harmony with the universe; it is necessary that everything with which he is concerned, or anything that is in his environment, is in full alliance and harmony with the Cosmic Structure and its basis in Cosmic Intelligence.

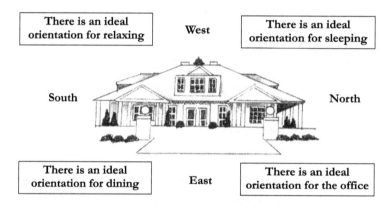

Sthapatya Veda is that aspect of cosmic knowledge of Natural Law which maintains the buildings in which the individual lives and works, and the environment in which he moves, well set in cosmic harmony.[54]

Today, many of us are at least partially aware of the ways that our environments affect us mentally and physically. We know that pollutants, pesticides and toxins in our water and food and the air we breathe are taking their toll on our health. Health officials work to rid buildings of asbestos and lead-based paints, and the EPA estimates

---

54 Maharishi Mahesh Yogi, "Celebrating Perfection in Administration," 1998

that up to seventy million people may get sick because of harmful conditions in the workplace. Toxic construction materials, faulty air circulation and filtering systems and production chemicals have all been recognized as environmental toxins.

However, fewer people are aware that a building's design and its placement on a given site are equally potent health factors. Sthapatya Veda is an ancient system of architecture and town planning that supports alignment with Natural Law. According to architect Jonathan Lipman, a national expert on Frank Lloyd Wright, in Vedic architecture we find "a series of principles which describe the fine mechanisms whereby nature creates proportion and shapes objects, such as planets and stars and trees and human bodies. This ancient discipline of Sthapatya Veda gives us these principles and allows architects to apply them to creating houses and office space. And when we do that-and when people live in these buildings-they have the most profound experience of „being at home' because they are in an environment that is entirely consistent with their own inner nature."[55]

The purpose of Vedic architecture is to bring the inhabitants of any building into alignment with Natural Law, as it is expressed both locally and universally. When the buildings in which we live and work are out of alignment with both local and universal values of Natural Law, we find ourselves swimming against the current, just as when the flow of our activity strains against natural cycles. The result can be anything from sickness to financial loss to family crises or all

---

55 "Making a House a Home," Enlightenment, Vol. 2, Issue 2, op. cit., P.38.

round "bad luck." I use quotes here, because bad luck can be understood as lack of support from the laws of nature. When we violate an aspect of Natural Law, when some area of life has lost its alignment with the flow of the universe, then the laws of nature which govern that flow will not back our efforts. We can find ourselves working hard and still experiencing negative results or falling ill.

One of the most important factors in Sthapatya Veda is called vastu, which means "holistic structure of Natural Law." Vastu incorporates a detailed consideration of the relationship among a building, its site and the local and distant environments. An ideal building location will bring positive influences from the sun, moon and each planet. It creates conditions in which every activity in a home or office can be in harmony with the cosmos. Improper vastu generates mental, physical, emotional or financial strain or even crisis. Proper vastu promotes ease and health in all areas of life

The determination of a proper vastu involves three main considerations:

1. Correct Orientation. A building's relationship to the movements of the sun is the most important factor. When your home or office faces east and your front door opens to the rising sun, your brain functions at its best. The sun's energy is at its maximum as it rises and that vitality is most available via an east entrance. A northern entrance is also helpful, but all other directions can produce stress or misfortune.

If your body is not facing in the optimum direction as you enter your home or perform activity, the brain's neuronal activity is actually inhibited. Recent biological research supports this ancient knowledge. It shows that the electrical activity in the thalamus shifts when the body changes its orientation, whether it's in a room or outdoors.

In addition to orientation to the sun, building placement involves evaluation of a lot's slope and shape, the existence and position of bodies of water, location of roads or streets and the elements and layout of the landscape-gardens, wooded areas, hills, etc. Instructions for the best arrangement of furniture and appliances are also given.

2. Correct Placement. We receive different qualities of the sun's light, warmth and energy as it moves through the sky each day. Each room of a building should be situated so that its activity benefits from the appropriate value of the sun's gifts, and Vedic architecture gives placement instructions for every room according to its function. The kitchen, for instance, needs maximum sunlight to provide the energy for cooking and is placed in the southeast corner of a house. When rooms are incorrectly located, it causes errors and stress. A wrongly placed bedroom might result in insomnia or too much sleep; a poorly located office might result in bad decisions or poor productivity.

3. Correct Proportion. Maharishi Sthapatya Veda provides detailed mathematical formulas to determine the size of every wall, door, window and room. It also calculates the size of each room in relationship to the house as a whole and the size of the building in relationship to its site. The proportions of every building and room embody principles which align the building and its inhabitants with the cosmos.

Maharishi Sthapatya Veda applies these same principles to town planning. Imagine a community in which every building and every aspect of its design fostered health and life-supporting behavior on an individual and collective level. Imagine a community whose very layout optimized brain function, generated bliss and prevented disease. No. This is not your own personal equivalent of Disneyland. It is the real possibility offered by this ancient system of architecture. The knowledge is there, right down to the tiniest mathematical formula, just waiting to be used.

Maharishi Vedic City is a city in Jefferson County, Iowa, United States. The city was first incorporated in 2001. Vedic City, Iowa became the first city in the world to be built according to principles of ancient Vedic architectural design, aimed at creating greater health, happiness, and prosperity for its residents. It is based entirely on the ancient principles of Maharishi Sthapatya Veda design and other aspects of Maharishi Vedic Science.

Chapter Twelve

Prevention

With the Maharishi Ayur-Veda Pulse Diagnosis, the soul of the vaidya [Ayurvedic physician] connects and enters into the soul, the atman, of the patient. It connects at this level, the level of all life, and gets thrilled. It's like a sutra; it's like transcending; the thrill rises up. Then the heart and mind are filled with such welling-up of emotions and love and affection for the patient and that love is like the love of a mother for her child; she automatically knows what the cry of the child represents. On the ground of that balanced consciousness of the vaidya in the great love for the patient, the vaidya detects the imbalance and immediately prescribes the remedy. By this means the vaidya never gets tired; he is drawn to his patients; he gains from them. Just as the teacher gains more than the student, the vaidya gains more than the patient.[56]

Maharishi Mahesh Yogi (India, 1986)

The Amazing Art of Nadi Vigyan

A small corner of New Delhi called East Nizamuddin looks and feels more like an Indian village than a big city neighborhood. Bicycles and cars weave their way around cows and oxcarts in the dirt roadways and women cook over dung fires in the street. In a niche of this small colony, one of India's greatest human treasures, Dr. Brihaspati Triguna, practices Ayurvedic medicine in humble quarters. Every day, hundreds of people, with every imaginable medical condition, sit

---

56 "Maharishi Ayur-Ved Pulse Diagnosis," Maharishi Ayur-Veda Physician Training Course I, Maharishi Ayur-Veda Medical Association, 1993, p. 44.

quietly on the hard wooden benches in his waiting room, fanning themselves to get relief from the heat and flies. Dr Triguna usually manages to see and help all of them. They approach him one-by-one and he places three fingers on their wrists. In just seconds, he gives them a comprehensive and highly accurate picture of what is happening in their minds and bodies. With few words, he describes their doshic constitution; their dominant mental quality (sattwa, rajas or tamas); any doshic imbalance or toxic buildup which is currently causing illness or might do so in the future; and a list of tissues and organs that have some weakness or disease. His assistant scribbles rapid notes, trying to catch each observation. Then Dr, Triguna prescribes exactly the right herbs, choosing from the thousands available without reference to any written list. He does not charge for his services.

Dr. Triguna is India's top practitioner of the astoundingly accurate art of nadi vigyan, or pulse diagnosis. Pulse diagnosis is one of the great jewels of Ayurvedic medicine. Though it takes considerable training and practice to gain the necessary sensitivity and clarity, nadi vigyan provides detailed and reliable information on a patient's condition. It tells which doshas and subdoshas are out of balance; the quality and strength of the digestive fire; where and how much ama has accumulated; which tissues and organs are affected; which stage of disease a patient is experiencing; the patient's doshic constitution.

This thorough printout of a patient's physiology is invaluable in showing me the deepest causes of hi or her condition. Arthritis is such a complex disease and has so many secondary symptoms, which could arise as a result of any number of factors. I am so grateful for a diagnostic tool that almost invariably spotlights the primary pathogenic imbalances. With this input, I can treat my patients with confidence.

Too often, I see patients who are feeling confused, hopeless or misunderstood. Allopathic medicine has been unable to relieve their pain and their doctors have run out of alternatives. Jenna, for instance, was a thirty-seven-year-old painter and sculptor, who had been told she was a hypochondriac when her doctors could not understand or treat her complaints. This evaluation only made her feel anxious and depressed. As an artist who also loved gardening, Jenna used her hands a lot and this is where she started to feel occasional pain. The pain spread to her shoulders, then her neck, upper back and ankles. It eventually increased in frequency until it began to affect her every day. She also had a number of chronic conditions: sinus problems, allergies and migraine headaches two or three times per week. Her doctor prescribed medication for her headaches, joint pain and allergies, but said that she did not have arthritis. He could not locate the cause of the joint pain.

The prescriptions irritated Jenna's stomach and produced heartburn and acid reflux, as well as acne all over her body. She also developed sleep problems. When she returned to her doctor, she was labeled a hypochondriac and put on anti-depressant and sleep medication. This brought on severe PMS, which would last up to two weeks and produce anger and aggressiveness. On a friend's recommendation, Jenna finally decided to try Maharishi Vedic Medicine. Through nadi vigyan and MVM's other precise diagnostic tools, I was able to determine that Jenna did indeed have a significant imbalance and to treat it appropriately with diet and herbs. Within one month, Jenna's joint pain was resolved and her acid reflux, heartburn and indigestion had also been corrected. She stopped using painkillers, sleep medicine and the many over-the-counter supplements she had been trying. After three more months, almost every initial symptom had been relieved, including her headaches. As a bonus, Jenna also lost eight pounds, which she loved. Not all joint pain is arthritis or degenerative and Jenna's doctor was correct in saying that arthritis was not her problem, at least not yet. Remember that Ayurveda describes six stages of disease. Symptoms like pain, headaches and chronic congestion are a clear message from our bodies that something is wrong. If we do not pay attention to the early signals of imbalance, then almost inevitably, full-blown diseases such as FMS or OA will develop in time, especially when we enter the vata-dominant stage of life.

Personal Preventive Measures

A number of the most widespread forms of arthritis involve an inherited predisposition to develop the disease, e.g., rheumatoid arthritis, gout, ankylosing spondylitis and possibly lupus. Due to the increase of vata dosha, as we age, everyone is a candidate for osteoarthritis. Fortunately, we do not all get sick, so we know that these conditions are not inevitable, irrespective of our genetic makeup. However, since we know the potential is there, why not choose to live in a way that minimizes the possibility of illness?

To maintain healthy digestion and doshic balance, try to see an MVM physician seasonally to determine your doshic constitution and any current imbalances. If you have occasional, mild discomfort, don't let it continue. It's not just the weather. It's the weather exacerbating your own doshic disequilibrium. Once clear disease symptoms appear, the imbalance, as you now know, is well-established and more difficult to reverse. Make the changes in your diet and lifestyle that will restore health long before conditions become chronic. Follow the diets, herbs and other recommendations of your MVM physician; follow the daily and seasonal routines that keep you moving in harmony with Natural Law.

You can even learn nadi vigyan yourself to benefit you and your family. Early in this book, I mentioned that one of the goals of MVM is to make people self-sufficient in their healthcare. If you develop the ability to read the pulse for yourself and close family members, you can make pulse diagnosis a standard part of your family's health care. You will be able to detect imbalances just as they arise, on a daily basis, and correct them immediately, often just through adjustments in your diet or routine.

I had a lupus patient who learned pulse diagnosis through the course offered by Maharishi Vedic University.[57] During one office visit, she told me: "When you touch me and take my pulse, I feel calmer right away." I told her that she could do the same thing-and she did. In fact, she became excellent at discerning her own imbalances. Whenever her pulse reading pointed to the start of doshic imbalance, she

---

[57] The Appendix provides information on the university and other resources that I have mentioned.

applied the knowledge about diet, oil massage and other therapies that MVM gave her.

She had suffered from lupus for almost fifteen years, but after starting on an MVM treatment regimen, she no longer had to use steroids. She took the time to take care of herself and made good progress even in the midst of an extremely demanding and stressful work life.

Maharishi Jyotish: Averting Danger Before It Arises

Just as we are affected on a daily and seasonal basis by the cycles of the sun and moon, we are also affected by the cycles of the other planets in our solar system. Throughout human history, almost every culture has had some method of tracking the movements of the planets and their influence. The Vedic Literature provided the original astrological system, called jyotish, which Maharishi defines as the science of transformation and the technology of prediction. Maharishi Jyotish is based on the sequential unfoldment of creation from pure consciousness, which the Veda describes and embodies. Maharishi Jyotish takes this knowledge of how cosmic intelligence unfolds creation from the unified field and applies it to the art of prediction. Jyotish encompasses the understanding of how all life evolves from underlying wholeness. Therefore it also contains the knowledge of how any individual life unfolds through time.

Physics depicts the emergence of the physical world from the unified field as a predictable and orderly process, which parallels the Vedic portrait of creation. Whether we look at physics or the Veda, we see that creation takes place in a definite progression. If we think of a car factory, or any production line that builds something, it does so in a fixed sequence. If someone knows that sequence, he or she can inspect the product at any point in the line and know which steps have been completed and which remain to be done. Similarly, each human life is in production. Maharishi Jyotish provides detailed mathematical formulas that allow a trained expert to "inspect" any point in an individual's life. He or she can tell which steps or events have passed and which are yet to come and when they will occur.

Your birth chart is like a cosmic snapshot. It encompasses all the planetary movements and influences at the moment you were born. Think of the planets and stars as laws of nature whose attributes and interactions provide a kind of blueprint for your life. The planets, or grahas, are much more than large bodies in the heavens. They are influences that permeate nature, including our own mind/body. They are such an intimate part of us that we can think of them as our cosmic counterparts.

The natal chart, or janma kundali, is divided into twelve houses that describe the major categories of experience, including wealth, relationships, spiritual development and health. The position of the grahas in these houses, which is determined based on the time and place of birth, gives information which can be extremely useful in helping prevent disease. The kundali describes your mental, emotional and physiological strengths and weaknesses. Progressed through time using detailed calculations, the chart will show when health-related events, such as disease, accidents or general weakness,

Prevention

will arise and what mental or physical aspects of your life will be affected.

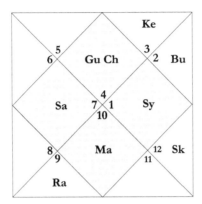

If someone is already ill, the chart will identify the celestial influences that led to the problem. It can point to the exact cause and nature of any medical condition. When the root cause of disease is accurately defined, it can be treated with the greatest effectiveness. If the seed of disease lies in future conditions, steps can be taken to prevent it.

For example, if you knew that a propensity for gout ran in your family and that it generally showed up around age thirty, you could take proper preventive measures, such as changing your diet and lowering your stress levels long before that time. Similarly, if your chart showed a predisposition for rheumatoid arthritis and that the tendency for RA would get exacerbated at a certain point in time, you could act beforehand to minimize those pathogenic influences.

In addition to all the options that Maharishi Vedic Medicine offers to facilitate balance and prevention, Maharishi Jyotish also provides some preventive and remedial measures. Maharishi Yagyas, the most important of these measures, are traditional procedures performed by specially trained Vedic pundits in India before a difficult or dangerous event or condition arises. These ancient procedures both neutralize negative influences so that they do not reach the individual and enhance individual success. If sickness has already manifested, Maharishi Yagyas can counteract the causes and maximize the effectiveness of medical treatments. Though usually done for an individual, these powerful performances also enliven Natural Law for the benefit of society as a whole.

The value of knowing the future is to be able to do some thing about it. Maharishi Jyotish sheds light on the road ahead so that we can avert problems and take advantage of opportunities coming our way. We have so many opportunities to reconnect with wholeness and realign ourselves with Natural Law. I encourage you to take action and indulge in some healthy changes to ensure a vital future.

Chapter Thirteen

Pulling Everything Together: The End of this Book-and Joint Disease

The purpose of a science of living, if it is to be a perfect science of living, is to make the individual breathe cosmic existence, to allow him to live the totality of universal life within all the boundaries of living. This is accomplished by attuning to that field where all the laws of nature are wide awake, the home of all the laws of nature.

-*Maharishi Mahesh Yogi*[58]

Joan was in her late forties and experiencing pre-menopausal symptoms when she came for her first MVM consultation. She had had water retention, joint stiffness and pain before her periods and recently this had become worse. She now felt stiffness and pain in her joints during as well as before menstruation. After a few months on the Ayurvdic regimen which I recommended, she was much better and remained so.

She reported, "I realize how important every aspect of Ayurveda is, how everything is complete and wholesome-food, herbs, oil massage, the TM technique, panchakarma. They have a great value in themselves, and all together they are extremely effective in combating chronic problems." Joan's observation is important. MVM is a complete program for healthcare, not just a single herb here or there. It is not a network of bandaids, but rather a deep,

---

[58] Maharishi Mahesh Yogi, "Keynote Address," Science, Consciousness and Aging, MERU Press, West Germany, 1990, p. 13.

lasting and comprehensive healing system. Many options are available, as you have seen, and they work together synergistically, but the system is also flexible. I often start my patients with simple changes, a few herbal compounds, exercise and some dietary changes. I let them see how they feel and decide how far they want to go.

I know that strain will defeat the healing process. I also know that as my patients become healthier and more balanced, their newly-enlivened biological intelligence will become their guide. If they eat something wrong, their bodies will know, and they will be sensitive to the signals. The physician is the initial guide, but then the patient's inner intelligence takes over and right choices become automatic.

I have tried to accompany the description of each MVM recommendation and treatment with a basic understanding of its origin and purpose, chapter by chapter, because I know that a little knowledge can go along way towards inspiring healthy choices. However, in the name of wholeness and to make them simpler to follow, I would now like to consolidate the various treatment recommendations for you in one place.

A number of factors are common to all the treatment regimens for arthritis. In each case, for instance, practice of the TM and TM-Sidhi programs will be extremely helpful. These practices overcome pragyaparadha, that disconnection from Nature's infinite intelligence that is the ultimate cause of all disease. They help restore the memory of perfect function at a cellular and system level and enliven biological intelligence and the mind/body's capacity for self-healing.

They dramatically decrease stress, which plays such a strong role in vata-related diseases. They also open every level of life-mental, physical, emotional-to bliss, which is a marvelous gift to anyone, but especially someone in pain.

With the exception, perhaps, of carpal tunnel syndrome, the first approach to healing all of the conditions we have described is what Ayurveda calls amapachana, the dissolution and elimination of ama. In most conditions, but especially amavat (RA), if we do not do this first, nothing else will be very effective. To facilitate the meltdown and removal of ama, I recommend sipping hot water throughout the day. In addition, follow the general guidelines for eating in Chapter Eight, as well as the ideal dinacharya or daily routine. Eat a light, nourishing diet which pacifies the appropriate dosha. Emphasize warm, well-cooked food and warm beverages. If agni is weak, your doctor may recommend that you start with soupy, liquified foods and progress gradually toward a normal diet.

Osteoarthritis. Follow the diet to pacify kapha and vata, but emphasize kapha at first. When agni is rekindled, focus more on vata. Artichokes and asparagus are excellent. Use digestive spices: ginger, cumin, turmeric, cloves, fenugreek, garlic, pepper. Emphasize bitter and pungent food and spices.

Spondylitis. Follow a vata- and kapha-pacifying diet, as above.

Rheumatoid Arthritis and Lupus. Emphasize bitter and pungent foods and spices, especially ginger. Physician-supervised fasting can also help. Avoid all heavy proteins and heavy, oily food in general, including rich proteins like meat and cheese. Avoid eating foods in the wrong combinations-with contradictory virya (potency), for example. (See Chapter Eight.) Cook with cumin, ginger, turmeric and cloves. Since RA can involve all three doshas, the doshic emphasis for diet will have to be prescribed by your MVM physician after diagnosis.

Fibromyalgia. Emphasize a light, vata-pacifying diet. Avoid sour, spicy, salty food. Gout. Both vata and pitta must be pacified. Avoid hot, sharp, sour, pungent and fermented food, including alcohol, caffeine, vinegar and soy sauce. Avoid rich proteins (meat, poultry, cheese, eggs) and oily, heavy food. Decrease salt intake. Use olive oil and avoid sesame oil. Eat green, leafy vegetables, especially fennel.

Carpal Tunnel Syndrome. Eat to pacify both vata and kapha. Maharishi Rejuvenation Therapy is a powerful aid for eliminating ama as well as balancing the doshas. Maharishi Rejuvenation Therapy often includes a series of treatments for each condition, though they must be individually prescribed by an MVM physician.

For osteoarthritis: abhyanga, swedana, basti, pinda swedhana (especially for hips and knees), baluka swedhana (fomentation treatment with sand), pizzichilli, shirodhara

For spondylitis: abhyanga, pizzichilli, pinda swedhana

For rheumatoid arthritis and lupus: abhyanga (after the ama has been reduced through diet and herbs); swedana, pinda swedhana, pizzichilli, shodhana basti

For fibromyalgia: abhyanga, shirodhara, pizzichilli, pinda swedana, shodhana basti

For gout: abhyanga, virechana, pinda swedhana

For carpal tunnel: abhyanga, pinda swedhana

Additional Recommendations

Osteoarthritis

- Daily abhyanga with sesame oil or Maharishi Ayur-Veda herbalized oil for vata (Herbal Massage Oil Moisturizing), emphasizing the joints
- Herbs: Joint Soothe 1 and 2, Maharishi Ayur-Veda Herbal Cleanse, triphala. ashwanganda, Maharishi Ayur-Veda Amala-Berry, Maharishi Ayur-Veda Calcium Rich, castor oil
- Regular routine, especially going to sleep on time.

Spondylitis

- Use a gentle, but regular exercise routine to keep joints flexible. If the disease is not too advanced, use asanas, properly learned, to help prevent further damage. Here are the names of a few which are often recommended: chetasana, kathiasana, hastpadasana, shalabasana, janushirasana.
- Maintain proper posture, whether walking or sitting at work. Keep your spine relaxed but straight, and don't bend or lift from the lumbar spine.
- Give yourself a daily abhyanga with sesame oil or Maharishi Ayur-Veda herbalized oil for vata (Herbal Massage Oil Moisturizing).
- Herbs: Joint Soothe 1 and 2.

Rheumatoid Arthritis and Lupus

- Daily abhyanga after the ama has been eliminated.
- Herbs: Castor oil, senna, triphala, Joint Soothe 1 and 2.
- Gentle exercise for the joints, which involve flexion and extension; swimming and asanas (properly learned), including:

chetasana, vajrasana, padmasana, shukhasna, sun salutation.
- Shukhpranayam
- Maharishi Ayur-Veda Aroma Oils F, L, M.
- If RA is just in the beginning stages, then even a change in diet will help in a few weeks and provide significant change in a few months. However, if the disease is chronic and well-established, the recommendations may have to become a permanent lifestyle.
- Eat a light dinner, no later than 6 or 6:30 PM. Morning stiffness is due to kapha and this will help decrease the stiffness. Eat light grains, like couscous, or soupy vegetables, dahl.

Fibromyalgia Syndrome

Along with amapachana and reinvigorating digestion, the treatment of FMS must include measures to decrease stress and strengthen the nervous system. Regular practice of the TM technique is of great value here.

- Herbs: Ashwaganda, triphala, Maharishi Ayur-Veda AmalaBerry and Joint Soothe 1 and 2, brahmi and other herbs to reduce mental stress and relax the muscles, mahanarayana oil.
- Maharishi Ayur-Veda Slumber Time and Worry Free Tea.
- Massage the feet before bed with ghee or olive oil.
- Daily abhyanga with Maharishi Ayur-Veda Herbal Massage OilMoisturizing (for vata)
- Yoga asanas, properly learned: chetasana, vajrasana, shavasana, sashankasana, sun salutations.
- Shukhpranayama, properly learned.

Gout
- Get enough sleep and maintain an active, involved, but not pressured, lifestyle.

- Practice the TM technique to decrease stress and anger.
- Herbs: Maharishi Ayur-Veda Liver Care, Acid Balance, Rejuvenation Oil, Maharishi Ayur-Veda AmalaBerry.
- Maharishi Ayur-Veda Aroma Oil G.
- Do a ghee-based virechana (cleansing) treatment monthly. See your MVM physician for details.

Carpal Tunnel Syndrome

- To prevent or help reduce carpal tunnel syndrome, adopt measures that save your wrists. If your work involves repetitive motion, including computer work, take breaks. Exercise your hands, fingers and wrists, using rotation, flexion and extension movements.
- Massage your wrists and hands with Maharishi Ayur-Veda herbalaized kapha and vata oil (Herbal Massage OilStimulating and Moisturizing).
- Use pinda swedana treatments for the wrists. These are available as part of Maharishi Rejuvenation Therapy.
- Herbs: Joint Soothe 1 and 2.

In Case You Still Have Questions

I have been a doctor long enough to be able to hear your questions and hesitations even before you speak them out. You have read the explanations and case histories and seen the scientific evidence, but perhaps still feel some reluctance, some disbelief. Maybe it sounds too good to be true; or maybe it is just a very long stretch between your prior understanding of medicine and Ayurveda. Let me see if I can allay some of your doubts.

1. Will MVM work for me?

This system of medicine is for everyone and for every day. It helps dissolve all kinds of joint pain, even joint pain that is not from arthritis. It is also helpful at any stage of the disease process, from early to advanced. In fact, it is good even if no disease is present and you want to prevent illness.

2. What if I am taking conventional medicine? Will MVM still work?

Conventional medicine is fine until your MVM treatment brings relief from the symptoms. This could take a few days or a few weeks. Then we can gradually wean you from the conventional prescriptions.

3. I am using MVM and I have 80 to 90 percent relief. What can I do about the discomfort that still remains?

Depending on your discomfort threshold, you could try a little over-the-counter medicine like Tylenol or Motrin.

4. What are the chances of a cure?

In my experience, the early stages of joint pain and arthritis are all curable. In the later stages, you can expect longer remissions, an improved quality of life, the prevention of additional degeneration and a substantial reduction in the need for conventional medicines.

5. How does the MVM treatment regimen differ from that of conventional medicine?

With conventional treatment, you will typically be put on a pain killer and then progress to anti-inflammatory agents. If your condition is still unmanageable, you will be given steroids and immuno-suppressants. This is currently standard for all patients. In MVM, we recognize that each patient is different and we prescribe treatments based on the uniqueness of each patient's physiology. This greatly enhances the chance for cure, long-lasting relief or lengthy remissions.

6. The program appears complex and time-consuming. Can I handle it?

If patients have a lot of pain or fatigue, I start them off with simple recommendations and small dietary changes-things they can handle until they feel better. Then I add other therapies gradually so that they are not overwhelmed. Please understand that MVM is extremely flexible. There is nothing rigid about its protocol. Of course, when you add more therapies, the pace of healing quickens. However, you should never strain to take on more than you can handle. Strain only creates more weakness. I work carefully with my patients to achieve the best treatment program for them.

7. How long do I need to use MVM?

MVM has to be used for a long time in most cases of joint disease. Some MVM therapies should be used every day; e.g., diet, oil massage, the TM technique and yoga postures. Herbs are usually given at the start of the treatment regimen, but many patients have gone completely off the herbs and maintained a long remission. In chronic disease, however, we usually recommend that certain herbs-perhaps one or two-be used on a continuous basis.

8. If I study Ayurveda and self-select herbs from a catalogue or health food store, will I benefit?

Gaining knowledge plays an important role in correcting pragyaparadh (the intellect's mistaken identity with the objective world rather than its unbounded source) and guiding us in the direction of healthy diet and lifestyle choices. However, the treatment of most forms of joint disease is quite complex. We find so many secondary symptoms: swelling, numbness, fluid accumulation, weight gain, skin problems, constipation, digestive and sleep disorders, fatigue, anxiety and depression to name a few. Even the nature of patients' pain may differ due to doshic dominance-vata vs. pitta. All these factors have to be considered so that you don't end up going to a dozen specialists and taking a dozen prescriptions.

The correct MVM herbs can address and relieve a whole complex of symptoms. They produce balance, and do not disturb the elements or tissues or have harmful side effects. They create health and longevity in addition to impacting disease. However, one has to have training to match the patient's special needs with the right set of herbs and to understand their unique medicinal qualities. Consequently, many of the MVM herbal formulas are only available from a trained physician, as opposed to a catalogue or health food store. Remember that all the MVM formulas come from the ancient science of dravyaguna.. Their use is precisely defined and they are prepared meticulously by traditional methods.

9. How does MVM compare with other forms of natural medicine?

This could be a long answer, but I feel that the most important thing to mention is that MVM enlivens wholeness. Its therapies deal not only with the most concrete expressions of disease, but also with its deepest and subtlest cause-the disconnection from consciousness, from our own essential nature. We not only eradicate disease and its symptoms, but also reestablish balance at every level of the mind and body.

When we create health through MVM, we create something very big. Our goal is Bliss, in our awareness and in our bodies. MVM uses the most ancient and powerful technologies available to return each human being to his birthright: life lived at the highest levels of inner and outer fulfillment.

Ayurveda: A Compassionate Science

Sharon had bilateral carpal tunnel syndrome, which she blamed on too much computer time. She came to see me after having surgery on her right side. A few weeks after the surgery, scar tissue had developed, and a short time later, pain tingling and numbness . returned and got worse. After six weeks, her doctors told her that surgery would have to be repeated and they could not guarantee success.

She came to MVM as last resort, but after a few weeks of treatment, pain had decreased in both her arms. Within two months, her discomfort had decreased by 80 percent and she felt that she no longer needed surgery. Two years later, she continues to enjoy good health.

Jack, a male patient in his mid-forties, had muscle pain and arthralgia (pain without swelling) when he came for help. He had not responded well to conventional medicine. Within a few months of Ayurvedic treatment, his problem was completely gone.

A woman in her early thirties, named Deborah, had RA, with swelling and pain in the small joints of her hand and feet as well as in her knees, elbows and shoulder. Her pain was so great that she had difficulty doing even simple household tasks. Her disease had begun in her twenties, then become more severe after pregnancy. She had tried steroids and NSAIDs but feared their long term side effects. She had also tried homeopathy and various herbs but experienced only marginal improvement.

After a few weeks on an MVM regimen, she felt relief and continued to progress quickly. She has maintained a healthy lifestyle suitable to RA prevention-including panchakarma therapy twice a year-over the last five years. She has remained free of swelling and pain. When I last saw her, she was feeling really alive. Her life had become rich. She could take care of her family and do more than ever before.

I have many more stories like this that I could share with you. It is both humbling and gratifying to find a system of medicine that takes people from an existence dominated by disease to a life which is better than ever before.

No one is more aware of the suffering pervading modern life than those in the healing professions. We see this irrespective of the breakthroughs of modern science and technology and the external forms of comfort we have created for ourselves. We keep spending millions of dollars on research to find cures for the many diseases that plague us, yet the solution is already available and very old indeed.

Try to imagine how thrilled I was when I began to study MVM and use it in my medical practice. I finally had access to a healthcare system that was powerful and pervasive in its effects, not only healing painful and complex illnesses but also redefining health in terms of the fullest values of human happiness and potential.

Maharishi Vedic Medicine supplies what has been lacking in modern science and medicine-an integrated and unifying perspective. Ayurvedic medicine begins and ends with wholeness, the unified field of Natural Law. Every part of life is understood in terms of its origin in that wholeness as well as its relationship to every other part. Whereas allopathic medicine has brilliantly identified and analyzed individual areas of knowledge, its understanding of health exists in isolated bits and pieces. Despite the best intentions of doctors and researchers, the result is a dehumanized, high-tech medicine with too many unknown side effects.

Recently, Tony Nader, a medical doctor and Ph.D. working with Maharishi, discovered direct correspondences between the major components of the human brain and physiology and the structure of the Veda and Vedic Literature. In simplest terms, this means that we are structured in the same patten of intelligence as the physical universe. We are part of a great web of life, each part another beautiful expression of the same infinite wholeness; each thread fluctuating in perfect harmony with every other strand of the universe. When we are healthy, each cell performs its role perfectly and in perfect harmony with every other cell in our bodies every atom in the universe. Human beings are indeed cosmic.

When patients arrive in my office, no matter how much pain they have, I can meet them with a confidence and optimism that uplifts their spirits. To treat them, I must see them as unique individuals and thus they feel nurtured and accepted, rather than fearful and alone. Beyond that, I am fundamentally connected to each and everyone of them, for they are all a reflection of my own deepest nature. Maharishi Vedic Medicine is based in wholeness at every level, from the quality of its treatments to the compassion with which it is offered. I leave you with one last portrait of the possibilities for perfect health.

... But compassion and kindness are wide awake in a man who is happy, who is peaceful. Therefore we need not keep ourselves on the platform of suffering. This...gives us a stand on our own peace and happiness, and then more ability, greater compassion, kindness and all virtues appear. With that we maintain our peaceful surroundings, and wherever we go, we take the aura of peace and happiness. You attain a status in life whereby through every thought of yours, through every speech of yours, and through every action of yours, the whole creation will be helped without your trying to help.[59]

---

[59] Maharishi Mahesh Yogi, Thirty Years Around the World, Vol. 1, MVU Press, The Netherlands, 1986, p. 310.

INDEX

A

abhyanga 109, 159, 164, 172, 184, 214, 215, 216
accumulation 9, 101, 142, 143, 220
aggravation. 30, 119, 123, 135, 173, 185
agni 65, 90
akasha 65
ama. 94, 100
amrit Kalash 187
ankylosing spondylitis 31, 118
anupanas 183
apana Vata 74
aroma therapy 186
arthritis 15, 16, 17, 18, 22, 23, 24, 26, 28, 31, 34
asanas 163, 193, 215, 216,

B

bala 102, 103, 185
bastis 174
bhutagnis 91
bliss 89, 142, 199, 213

C

cancer 2, 188
carpal tunnel syndrome 11, 33, 34, 135, 144, 164, 213, 217, 221
charaka Samhita 136, 158
chhandas 51, 59
chronic fatigue 45, 89
consciousness 48

D

daily routine 157
dhatu agni 92
devata 51, 59
dhatus 92
diet 131
digestion 89
dinacharya 159
See also daily routine
disease 52
    six stages of 110

Index

disruption 98, 115
dissemination 111
doshas 66, 67, 68, 69, 73, 77, 78, 79, 82, 83

E
environmental toxins 196

F
fibromyalgia 2, 8, 11, 24, 25, 45, 93, 108, 214
fibromyositis 89
Fomentation 173
free radicals 23

G
ghee 135, 147, 150, 151, 153, 154, 155, 160, 171, 183, 216, 217
grahas 207
gunas 60, 61, 62

H
herbalized oils 162, 174, 185
herbs 134, 136, 138, 140, 171, 172, 173, 174, 175, 179, 180, 181, 182, 183
honey 136, 140, 147, 148, 150, 151, 156, 183
hot flashes 10, 11, 79,
hypertension 123
hypothyroid 78

I
immune system 18, 26, 27, 37, 40, 124
immunity 102, 126, 182, 187, 188
indigestion 122, 123, 127, 145, 204
insomnia 73, 81, 111, 120, 198

J
janma kundali 207
jatharagni 90, 93, 94
jyotish 206

K
kapha 66, 67, 71, 77, 78, 81, 83, 84,

L
lassi 147, 150, 151, 156
laws of nature........................... 48, 55, 159, 192, 197, 207, 211
localization.. 123
longevity 187, 220
lower back pain.. 57, 74

M
mahabhutas.. 64, 66, 68
maharishi mahesh yogi 1, 5, 49, 57, 157, 179, 190, 201
maharishi rejuvenation therapy...................................... 169
malas.. 89, 174
mamsavaha srotas 97
manifestation 19, 66, 124, 180
meditation 5, 85, 143, 159, 160, 176
mistake of the intellect 53, 143

N
nadi vigyan 202, 205
nasya... 173, 174
nature's intelligence 182

O
oil massage... 162
ojas... 102, 103, 104, 105, 154, 182, 187
osteoarthritis.. 16, 21, 214

P
pachaka pitta 75
panchakarma... 121, 211, 222,
See also maharishi rejuvenation therapy
pinda swedana... 173
pitta 66, 67, 75, 76, 79, 80, 81, 84
pizzichilli... 172
prabhava... 183
Prana... 73, 194
pranayama.. 163, 194
prithivi... 91
pulse diagnosis 205,
See also Pure consciousness
pulse diagnosis.. 201
purification 169, 171

Index

R
ragas 192, 193
rajas 61, 62, 63, 141, 202
rakta dhatu 127
rasa 92, 141
rasa dhatu 95, 96, 122
rasayanas 175, 185, 187
rheumatoid arthritis... 191,
ritucharya 169
 See also seasonal routine

S
samana vata 73
seasonal routine.. 169
 See also ritucharya
sesame oil.................... 150, 154, 159, 164, 172, 184, 186, 214, 215
shirodhara... 173
snehana 171
srotas .... , 95, 96, 98, 99
blockage 143
sthapatya Veda... 195
subdosha 74, 77, 116
 See also doshas
swedana.. 17

T
tamas.. 61, 62, 63, 141, 202
tanmatras 64
tissues 92
 See dhatus
TM-Sidhi program 176, 177
toxins 75, 81, 89, 138, 162, 172, 174, 184, 186, 195, 196,
 See also ama
 elimination of 104, 170, 193
 environmental..................................... 86, 138, 196

U
udana 73
udvartana 172

V
vastu 197

vata 66, 67, 69, 70, 73, 74
vayu 65
Vedic architecture 196, 198
vipaka 132, 183
virechana 174
virya 142, 145, 183, 214
vyana Vata 74

W
waste products 75, 96, 100, 101, 104,
See also malas

Y
yagyas 209
yoga 193, 216

Appendix

Sources for Information on Maharishi Vedic Approach to Health and Related Programs

How to locate a vaidya (ayurvedic expert) in your area
National Tour Center   1-641-209-1981

To contact Kumuda Reddy, M.D.
5009 Paducah road, College Park, MD 20740
www.allhealthyfamily.com
Ph.: 1-866-REDDYMD
1-301-474-2184

CENTERS OFFERING TREATMENT PROGRAMS IN MAHARISHI AYURVEDA

The Raj Maharishi Ayurveda Health Center and Spa 800-248-9050 or
Fairfield, Iowa 641-472-9580
Web site: www.theraj.com

The Maharishi Vedic Health Center 877-890-8600 or
Lancaster, Massachusetts 978-365-4549
Website: http://www.lancasterhealth.com/learn/

Maharishi Vedic Vibration Technology 800-431-9680
Web site: www.vedicvibration.com
E-mail: applications@vedicvibration.com

WHERE TO ORDER MAHARISHI AYUR-VEDA PRODUCTS AND HERBAL FORMULAS

Appendix

In the United States
Maharishi Ayurveda Products
International, Inc. (MAPI)
402 N. B Street
Fairfield, IA 52556
Web site: www.mapi.com

800-255-8332 or
719-260-55

In Canada
Maharishi Ayurveda Products Canada
Web site: www.mapicanada.ca/index.asp

Get 10% discount on mapi products by using the code HP-206-0309 on selected products - US and Canada orders only

QUICK REFERENCE GUIDE OF MAHARISHI AYURVEDA PRODUCTS THAT WOULD BE HELPFUL IN ARTHRITIS, FIBROMYALGIA, MUSCLE PAIN AND JOINT PAIN

For Muscle & Joint Problems

1. Osteo Relief
2. Spice Mix
3. Calcium Support
4. Joint Soothe tablets
5. Joint Soothe II oil

To Balance Digestion

1. Aci - balance
2. Digest Tone
3. Herbal Di- Gest

To Detox

1. Elim Tox
2. Elim Tox O
3. Herbal Cleanse
4. Genitrac
5. Mind Flex
6. Worry Free

To Help with Sleep

1. Deep Rest
2. Blissful Sleep
3. Slumber Time Tea
4. Slumber Time Aroma Oil

To Rejunvate the Liver

1. Liver Balance

For Energy & Vitality

1. Stress Free Body
2. ReGen Vitality
3. Vata Tea
4. Stress Free mind

For General Rejuvenation

1. Rejuvenation for Men
2. Rejuvenation for Ladies
3. Vital Lady
4. ReGen Vitality

To Improve Immunity

1. Bio - Immune
2. Amrit

To Help Balance the Mind & Emotions

1. Mind Plus
2. Stress Free Mind
3. Stress Free Emotions

Please ask Dr Reddy or call MAPI help line as to how to use these and other preparations. To get a 10% discount please use this code HP 206-0309.

TO LOCATE A TEACHER OF THE TRANSCENDENTAL MEDITATION TECHNIQUE IN YOUR AREA

Call toll-free 888-LEARN-TM (888-532-7686)
or see web site: www.tm.org.

FOR INFORMATION AND RESEARCH ON THE TRANSCENDENTAL MEDITATION TECHNIQUE

Information and research on the Transcendental Meditation Technique
www.tm.org

Doctors on the Transcendental Meditation technique and health benefits:
www.doctorsontm.org

The Transcendental Meditation technique and educational benefits:
www.tmeducation.org/
http://adhd-tm.org/

Appendix

Information for implementing and funding programs for teaching Transcendental Meditation in schools
www.davidlynchfoundation.org
www.cbeprograms.org/ (US)
www.consciousnessbasededucation.org.uk/ (UK)

MAHARISHI SCHOOLS AND UNIVERSITIES

Maharishi School of the Age of Enlightenment (For Children K-12)
In the United States:
804 North Third Street
Fairfield, IA 52556
866-472-6723
Fax: 641-472-1211
www.maharishischooliowa.org

Maharishi School of the Age of Enlightenment (For Children K-12)
In the United Kingdom:
Cobbs Brow Lane, Lathom
Ormskirk, Lancashire, L40 6JJ
UK
Phone: +44 (0)1695 729912
Fax: +44 (0)1695 729030
www.maharishischool.com

Maharishi University of Management
1000 N. 4th St.
Fairfield, IA 52557
(800) 369-6480 or (641) 472-1110
www.mum.edu/

HEALTH EDUCATION COURSES IN MAHARISHI AYUR-VEDA

Health Education Short Courses:
Full descriptions of these courses can be found at the following web site: www.Maharishi.org.

1. Human Physiology: Expression of Veda and the Vedic Literature
2. Good Health through Prevention
3. The Maharishi Yoga^{SM} Program
4. Self-Pulse Reading Course for Prevention
5. Diet, Digestion and Nutrition
6. Maharishi Vedic Astrology Overview
7. Maharishi Vedic Architecture

For training courses in Maharishi Ayur-Veda for physicians and other health professionals:
Maharishi Ayur-Veda Association of America
email: maaa@globalcountry.net
phone (877) 540-6222.

For Degree Programs in Maharishi Integrative Medicine:
Maharishi University of Management
Bachelor's degree and pre-med program
(800) 369-6480 or (641) 472-1110
E-mail: admissions@mum.edu
Web site: www.mum.edu/premed/

THE MAHARISHI VEDIC ASTROLOGY AND MAHARISHI YAGYA PROGRAMS IN THE UNITED STATES AND CANADA

Maharishi Vedic Astrology and Maharishi Yagya programs websites: www.maharishiyagya.org
            www.globalgoodfortune.com

For more information, choose the Time Zone you live in:
Time Zone 9 Eastern States (CT, DC, DE, FL, GA, MA, ME, MD, NJ, NC, NH, NY, OH, PA, RI, SC, VA, VT, WV)
530-877-8332 (phone) 530-327-7736 (fax)
maharishiyagyatz9@maharishi.net

Time Zone 10 Central States (AL, AZ, AR, CO, ID, IL, IN, IA, KS, KY, LA, MI, MN, MS, MO, MT, NE, NM, ND, OK, SD, TN, TX, UT, WI, WY)
503-639-0464 (phone) 503-639-3860 (fax)
maharishiyagyatz10@maharishi.net

Time Zone 11 Western States (AK, CA, HI, NV, OR, WA)
530-877-8332 (phone) 530-327-7736 (fax)
maharishiyagyatz11@maharishi.net

(**Outside the U.S.A. and Canada,** please contact the Maharishi Yagya program's international office in Switzerland at +4141-825-1525 phone, +4141-825-1526 fax, jyotish-yagya@maharishi.net email.)

MAHARISHI VEDIC ARCHITECTURE, MAHARISHI VASTU AND THE MAHARISHI STHAPATYA VEDA PROGRAM

Fortune Creating Homes and Communities
www.fortunecreatingbuildings.com
641-472-7570

Recommended Books

Books by Maharishi Mahesh Yogi

Life Supported by Natural Law. Washington, D.C.: Age of Enlightenment Press, 1986.

Maharishi Forum of Natural Law and National Law for Doctors. India:

Age of Enlightenment Publications, 1995.

Maharishi Mahesh Yogi on the Bhagavad-Gita: A New Translation and Commentary, Chapters 1-6. New York: Penguin Books, 1973.

Maharishi Vedic University: Introduction. India: Age of Enlightenment Publications, 1995.

Science of Being and Art of Living. New York: Penguin Books, 1995.

Scientific Research on Maharishi Vedic Approach to Health

Scientific Research on Maharishi's Transcendental Meditation and TM-Sidhi Program: Collected Papers, Volumes 16, available through Maharishi University of Management Press, Press Distribution, DB 1155, Fairfield, Iowa 52557.

Scientific Research on the Maharishi Transcendental Meditation and TM-Sidhi Programs: A Brief Summary of 500 Studies. Fairfield, Iowa: Maharishi University of Management Press, 1996.

Other Books

Nader, Tony, M.D., Ph.D. *Human Physiology: Expression of Veda and the Vedic Literature.* Vlodrop, The Netherlands: Maharishi Vedic University Press, 2001.

Deans, Ashely, Ph.D. *A Record of Excellence: The Remarkable Success of Maharishi School of the Age of Enlightenment.* Septermber, 2005.

Denniston, Denise. *The TM Book: How to Enjoy the Rest of Your Life.* Fairfield, Iowa: Fairfield Press, 1986.

Pearson, Craig, Ph.D. *The Complete Book of Yogic Flying.* Fairfield, Iowa: Maharishi University of Management Press, 2008.

Reddy, Kumuda, M.D., Egenes, Linda, and Mullins, Margaret, MSN,FNP. *For a Blissful Baby: Happy and Healthy Pregnancy through Maharishi Vedic Medicine.* Schenectady: New York. Samhita Productions, 1999.

Roth, Robert. *Maharishi Mahesh Yogi's Transcendental Meditation.* New York: Donald I. Fine, 1994.

Schneider, Robert, M.D., Total Heart Health: How to Prevent and Reverse Heart Diseasee with the Maharishi Vedic Approach to Health. Laguna Beach:CA. Basic Health Publications, 2006.

Wallace, R. Keith. The Neurophysiology of Enlightenment. Fairfield, Iowa: Maharishi International University Press, 1986.

Wallace, R. Keith. The Physiology of Consciousness. Fairfield, Iowa: Maharishi International University Press, 1993.

These books and others are available from
Maharishi University of Management Press   800-831-6523
Press Distribution DB 1155
Fairfield, Iowa 52557
E-mail: mumpress@mum.edu

Web site: www.mumpress.com/

A selection of books is also available from Maharishi Ayurveda Products International (see information above).

CPSIA information can be obtained
at www.ICGtesting.com
Printed in the USA
LVHW081604140719
624052LV00018B/550/P